Feast on Phytochemicals

Alkaloids

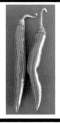 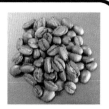

Betalains

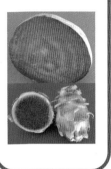

Phytosterols

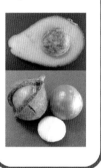

- Anti-inflammatory
- Antioxidants
- Balance cholesterol
- Brain stimulants
- Feed gut microbes
- Help prevent cardiovascular disease
- Help relieve depression
- Help reduce cancer risk
- Help with weight loss
- Lower blood pressure
- Protect our eyes
- Stimulate detox
- Relieve pain

Polyphenols

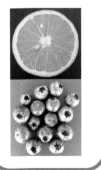

Sulphur compounds

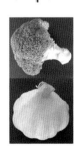

Terpenoids

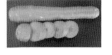

T0359707

Feast
on Phytochemicals

Natural health-boosting compounds
in fruit, vegetables, herbs and spices,
including Australian bush food plants

Paul R. Williams PhD

Feast on Phytochemicals. Natural health-boosting compounds in fruit, vegetables, herbs and spices, including Australian bush food plants.

by Paul R. Williams

Published by Vegetation Management Science Pty Ltd, Malanda, Australia © All rights reserved

For more information and to purchase a copy of this book please visit www.phytochemicalfeast.com

1st Edition 2019, paperback.

ISBN: 978-0-6484964-0-3

Cover design by Ryan McDonald-Smith and Julia Lefik
Cover photo by Eleanor Collins and Paul Williams
Book and text layout by Julia Lefik and Paul Williams
Edited and indexed by Sally Pope

Acknowledgements

I am extremely grateful to the many people who have helped me during the development of this book. I have benefited from discussions with many people, some of whom have also provided comments on earlier drafts. These people include Eleanor Collins, Dave Kington, Helen and John Hardman, Helen McConnell, Phoebe Pogorzelski, Kate Rogers, Terry Rose, Doug Unsworth, Diana Virkki, Phurpa Wangchuk, Alison and Isabelle Whitmill and Hans Wohlmuth. Sam and Kylie Collins at Blushing Acres avocado and mango farm provided valuable advice about horticultural issues. Sally Pope of SP Editing provided excellent editorial skills that improved the manuscript. Thanks also to Ryan McDonald-Smith and Julia Lefik for book and cover design assistance and Bruce Chaplin for printing advice. David Wilkinson, author of *Can Food be Medicine Against Cancer*, provided valuable discussions about the topic and advice about self publishing. I also thank James Cook University for providing access to scientific journals.

Disclaimer: The information contained within this book is for scientific and general educational purposes and discussion. It does not constitute medical or dietary advice, nor should it be seen as a replacement for that advice. The author is a plant scientist, with some biochemistry training (who grows fruit, vegetables, herbs and spices on his small property); not a medical doctor, nutritional scientist or dietician. While great care has been taken in researching and developing this book, neither the author or publisher accept any responsibility or liability for decisions or actions taken as a result of any information, statement or advice, expressed or implied, in this book. Readers should make their own detailed inquiries and obtain professional medical and dietary advice before making any decisions based on information contained in this book. All plants and plant products should be sourced from a reputable supplier, not from the wild.

Preface

Our passion for phytochemicals stretches back through millennia. Pharaohs were buried among them and Rome was ransomed with them. This obsession created global trade routes, was the reason for grand voyages of discovery and provided vast wealth to empires. The first significant shareholder corporations, the British and Dutch East India Companies, were created to unite investors in the trade of phytochemicals. That is, the spice trade.

Phytochemicals are chemicals made by plants (*phyto refers to plants, so phytochemicals = plant chemicals*). Phytochemicals are also known as phytonutrients. Of particular interest to this book are those that complement a plant's nutritional requirements, such as the caffeine in coffee beans. They are not the proteins, fats and sugars required for general plant (and human) growth, but are the countless chemicals plants manufacture to protect themselves from germs and herbivores, to attract pollinators and seed dispersers and to drive their hormone and enzyme systems.

Phytochemicals are the compounds that produce the kaleidoscope of colours that we see in fruit and vegetables. They are responsible for the brilliant flavours and medicinal properties of plants, including antioxidant and anti-inflammatory benefits that are critical to our health. They provide the pungent smell of garlic, the intense colour of blueberries, the zing of ginger and the heat of chillies. Phytochemicals include carotenoids in carrots, curcumin in turmeric and resveratrol in red wine.

The sophisticated chemistry that plants use to thrive provides compounds that are vital to our long-term health. Current research demonstrates that phytochemicals can help relieve the pain of arthritis, contribute to weight loss, and help reduce the risk of developing Alzheimer's disease, type 2 diabetes, heart disease, stroke and even some cancers. Phytochemicals can also boost healing and complement some medications.

This book does not promote a specific diet, beyond the encouragement to eat plenty of a variety of plants each day. It is advisable to always consult modern medical advice for illnesses and undertake appropriate treatments. The purpose of this book is to help explain why regularly eating a wide variety of minimally processed fruit, legumes, whole grains, nuts, vegetables, herbs and spices, as well as drinking tea and coffee and eating a small amount of dark chocolate, provides an essential contribution to good health.

Multiple lines of research demonstrate that if you are not eating a daily supply of at least two portions of fruit and five serves of vegetables, you're missing out on some amazing rewards. Every day that you do eat a colourful range of fruit and vegetables, and drink some tea or coffee, you are receiving help to reduce your blood pressure, clean your blood vessels, boost brain power, quench free radicals, remove toxins and reduce inflammatory pain.

Many of the phytochemicals in fruit, vegetables, herbs and spices provide health benefits through the same actions as common drugs, such as aspirin and anti-histamines, and when eaten in normal quantities, don't have the side effects that can be associated with many drugs. For example, cherries can help reduce gout symptoms, ginger can reduce inflammatory pain and nausea, cinnamon helps lower blood sugar levels, citrus fruit provide anti-histamines to help reduce hay fever symptoms. Drinking tea and eating dark chocolate can improve blood flow, reducing blood pressure by dilating blood vessels. Tea contains a phytochemical used in some asthma bronchodilator medications, while garlic and pomegranate can help reduce plaque formation in arteries. Eating plants of the cabbage and onion families, and the spice turmeric, can help reduce the chances of developing some cancers by assisting in the removal of carcinogens and inhibiting the growth of new blood vessels that supply nutrients to tumours. Many phyto-chemicals also promote beneficial gut bacteria.

In his book, *In Defence of Food*, Michael Pollan recommended eating whole food with little processing, mainly plants. This book is about those plants and the reasons they are so important to our health. It explores the role of phytochemicals in plants them-selves, and the results of some exciting new research showing how these plant compounds provide us with the health benefits that complement the flavours they provide.

Glossary of common terms and abbreviations used in this book

ALA stands for alpha-linolenic acid, which is an important omega 3 fat found in plants. It helps lower inflammation and our bodies convert a small proportion to other important omega 3 fats, EPA and DHA.

Angiogenesis is the process of growing new blood vessels around cells. It is involved in healing, and the growth of fat tissue and tumours.

Antioxidants stop the oxidising damage to our cells caused by compounds called free radicals. The browning of a sliced apple is an example of oxidation damage. Antioxidants work by giving up an electron to free radicals, but resist the temptation to steal an electron from another molecule, breaking the oxidation cycle. Many phytochemicals provide antioxidant benefits.

Atherosclerosis is the narrowing of blood vessels due to hardening and plaque build up. It contributes to heart attacks and strokes by limiting blood flow.

Carcinogens are compounds that can promote the development of cancer.

DHA refers to docosahexaenoic acid, which is a significant omega 3 fat found in fish, and smaller amounts in grass-fed livestock. A small proportion of ALA from plant sources converts to EPA and onto DHA. DHA plays an important role in our brain.

Enzymes are proteins that speed up chemical reactions in our bodies, ensuring important functions occur.

EPA stands for eicosapentaenoic acid, which is an important omega 3 fat, most abundantly found in fish. EPA helps reduce inflammation and blood clotting. A proportion of ALA from plant sources converts to EPA.

Free radicals are molecules within or around our cells that are unstable as a result of an unpaired electron. These free radicals are then compelled to steal an electron from another molecule, causing oxidative damage to proteins, DNA and fats, contributing to illnesses such as dementia and cardiovascular disease.

Glutathione is a powerful antioxidant made within our cells. It is produced in our bodies by combining three amino acids: cysteine, glutamic acid and glycine. Many phytochemicals stimulate the production of glutathione by activating a protein called Nrf2.

LDL stands for low density lipoprotein. As fats and cholesterol do not dissolve in water, and our blood is water-based, fats and cholesterol are transported within our blood in packets called lipoproteins. Lipoproteins range in size from very low density (VLDL) to high density (HDL). LDLs are often considered the 'bad' type of cholesterol. Research suggests it may not simply be the amount of LDLs in our blood that contributes to atherosclerosis, but whether they have been damaged by free radical oxidation, as well as the ratio of LDLs to HDLs.

Mitochondria are the energy producing units found in each cell.

Neurotransmitters are chemicals that transfer signals and messengers between nerves, including in the brain. Examples are dopamine and serotonin.

NF-kB is a type of protein called a transcription factor, found within our cells. When activated, particularly by our immune system, it triggers genetic information in our DNA to be used to produce inflammation-promoting compounds. These inflammation compounds include the enzyme cyclooxygenase 2 (COX-2), which catalyses the production of prostaglandin E2 from omega 6 fats.

Nrf2 is another transcription factor protein found within our cells. When Nrf2 is activated, such as by phytochemicals, it causes the translation of genetic information in our DNA to produce antioxidant compounds (especially glutathione).

Photosynthesis is the process by which plants use the energy from sunlight to combine water and carbon dioxide to produce sugar and oxygen.

Phytochemicals (also known as phytonutrients) are chemical compounds made by plants and are present in their bark, leaves, flowers fruit, roots and trunks. This book concentrates on phytochemicals not involved in primary plant growth (i.e. it does not focus on sugars, proteins and fats).

Placebo is the name given to a control treatment in a trial, which lacks the active ingredient. For example, a researcher may give half the participants in a trial a capsule containing turmeric powder and the other half a similar capsule containing no active ingredient (i.e. the placebo). The benefit of the turmeric powder is measured against any changes seen in people taking the placebo.

Superoxide dismutase (SOD), is a strong antioxidant made within our cells, in a similar fashion to glutathione.

Transcription factors are proteins within our cells, such as NF-kB and Nrf2, that transcribe genetic information in DNA, leading to the manufacture of compounds essential to our wellbeing.

A note about references *This book contains a review of nutritional and medical information, and therefore supplies a large reference list. This enables readers to examine the original study reports to develop their own interpretation of research results and to find further information. Throughout the text, studies and other books are referenced by referring to authors and the year of publication. This involves a standard format of author and year of publication, e.g. Wilkinson 2015. The source of these studies is found in the reference list at the back of the book, which is in alphabetical order of the first author's surname. The use of et al. indicates there were multiple authors, e.g. Konczak et al. 2012, refers to a study by Konczak and others, published in 2012.*

Table of Contents

Chapter 1
Introduction - Essential plant compounds

In June 1862, the Scottish-born Australian explorer John McDouall Stuart and his team were camped on the Roper River, near the present-day town of Mataranka in the Northern Territory. This was his sixth gruelling expedition into central Australia and it would become the first successful return crossing of the Australian continent by Europeans.

Stuart had a problem. At eight months into his journey he was suffering from scurvy. He wrote in his diary that he had 'scarcely been able to endure the motion of horseback for four hours at a time, but having lately obtained some native cucumbers, I find they are doing me a deal of good, and hope by next week to be all right again' (Stuart & Hardman 1865). Scurvy is a painful disease resulting from the degeneration of blood vessels and connective tissue. It is caused by a severe deficiency in a plant compound called ascorbic acid (vitamin C), as a result of not eating sufficient fruit or vegetables.

In October 1883, the Japanese ship *Riujo* returned to port after an absence of ten months. Echoing the devastation scurvy had wrought on European explorers, 169 of the 370 crew of *Riujo* were suffering from a disease known as beriberi. Twenty-five of the crew had died. A year later another Japanese ship, the *Tsukuba*, followed the same route as *Riujo*, but returned to Japan without a single case of beriberi. Having suspected diet was the cause of beriberi, a Japanese medical officer, Kanehiro Takaki, had arranged for the crew of the *Tsukuba* to eat meat and vegetables, in addition to their standard diet of mainly white rice (Itokawa 1976). In time, researchers discovered that beriberi is caused by a deficiency in a plant compound called thiamine (vitamin B1). This typically occurs when people eat mainly refined white rice, which loses its thiamine when the husk is removed during processing.

Today, the Japanese islands of Okinawa are home to some of the longest living people in the world and importantly, they maintain good physical and mental health into their old age (Buettner 2015). It is thought that one of the reasons the Okinawans are so healthy and active into old age is their diet rich in fish, fruit and vegetables (Willcox *et al.* 2014). Recent health problems in younger generations indicate that this longevity is not simply genetic, as many younger Okinawans are succumbing to increased rates of the same chronic diseases as people in western countries, such as cancer, heart disease and diabetes (Willcox *et al.* 2018). Many people in the younger generation have been eating a more westernised diet, with an increase in processed food and a decrease in fruit and vegetables (Buettner 2015). Is it possible that some of the younger generation of Okinawans are suffering from a deficiency in plant compounds?

Scurvy and beriberi are recognised as being caused by the lack of specific, essential chemical compounds made by plants, called vitamins. Yet a deficiency in the diversity of plant compounds, collectively called phytochemicals (meaning *plant-chemicals*), also known as phytonutrients, is probably common in people consuming modern western diets that lack a regular intake of a variety of fruit, vegetables, herbs and spices. This is sadly ironic, given that we in the developed world have easy access to such an abundance of available plant foods, and therefore phytochemicals, probably not seen before in human history.

Our appreciation of what is essential is relative to time. Hold your breath and you'll quickly recognise how essential oxygen is. Go without water in summer and you'll be keen for a drink within hours. Vitamins can take months to become noticeably deficient. It is probable that a range of phytochemicals are essential to the long-term maintenance of good health, but their absence may not become evident for many years. We can probably operate in a vaguely unhealthy state for years with low levels of phytochemicals.

We consume hundreds, even thousands, of different phytochemicals every time we feast on fruit and vegetables (including legumes and whole grains), herbs and spices. Phytochemicals are produced by plants to work as antioxidants, to activate their internal enzymes and hormones, defend themselves against being eaten, and to attract flower pollinators, fruit dispersers and symbiotic fungi to help them extract soil nutrients. Phytochemicals discussed in this book are those chemicals made by plants which do not directly contribute to growth. That is, this book does not focus on nutrients (proteins, fats and sugars) that are used as building blocks of cells or the fuel for energy, important as they are. It concentrates on the thousands of plant compounds that provide us with subtle yet essential health benefits, such as antioxidant and anti-inflammatory effects. You could think of phytochemicals as the pepper you sprinkle on your dinner. The pepper won't provide much in the way of nutrients for bone and muscle growth, but it provides the spice necessary for a good life.

Two examples of the many phytochemicals that are essential to our wellbeing are lutein and zeaxanthin. These compounds are found in numerous plants, such as avocado, carrots, corn, parsley and spinach, plus egg yolks (where they originate from the plants that chickens eat). They are absorbed into the cells of our eyes and are indispensable to eye health, with their antioxidant function inhibiting the development of macular degeneration and cataracts.

We are starting to grasp the idea that a range of phytochemicals are essential to us. Yet it is not a new idea. The Hungarian biochemist Albert Szent-Györgyi, who received the 1937 Nobel prize for research into vitamin C, argued that it worked best in synergy with another compound found in paprika and citrus. With his collaborator Professor Rusznyak, Szent-Györgyi determined this other compound to be an important group of phytochemicals called flavonoids, and proposed that they be considered essential, naming them vitamin P (Rusznyak & Szent-Györgyi 1936; Szent-Györgyi 1937).

Around 70 per cent of all deaths worldwide in 2015 were attributed to non-communicable diseases, especially cardiovascular disease, cancer and diabetes (World Health Statistics 2017). It is estimated that half of Australian adults suffer from a chronic disease (e.g. cardiovascular disease, cancer, dementia, depression, diabetes or inflammation such as arthritis), yet many instances of these diseases could be prevented with life style improvements (Tolhurst *et al.* 2016). A recent study estimated 38 per cent of cancer deaths in Australia during 2013 (that is 16,700 people) could have been prevented by life style changes, including increasing exercise, eating more fruit and vegetables and not smoking (Wilson *et al.* 2018). Contributing to these diseases is the fact that nearly two thirds of Australian adults, and about a quarter of children, are overweight and nearly a quarter of adults have high blood pressure (Tolhurst *et al.* 2016). This pattern is seen across much of the developed world.

There is consistent evidence that eating abundant fruit, vegetables, herbs and spices, plus drinking tea, is linked to a lower incidence of cardiovascular disease, some cancers, dementia, depression, type 2 diabetes, inflammation and Parkinson's disease. Our bodies respond well to eating a wide variety of plants, with some plant groups providing special value. Terry Wahls, an American doctor, has dramatically reduced her multiple sclerosis symptoms through a program that includes exercise, eliminating grains, legumes and dairy from her diet, while eating nine cups of fruit and vegetables a day. She is quite specific in her choices, ensuring she consumes a broad range of nutrients including valuable phytochemicals, with three of the nine cups from colourful fruit and vegetables and three from sulphur-containing vegetables, such as broccoli, garlic and onions (Wahls 2017).

Every plant provides a mix of phytochemicals. For example, coffee contains both alkaloids and polyphenols. Some of the most common plant foods we eat, such as oranges and tomatoes, provide extremely valuable phytochemicals. A few important phytochemicals are found in several plants, such as quercetin, which is a strong antioxidant and an inhibitor of inflammation with anti-histamine properties. Quercetin is present in many plants including apples, citrus, grapes, onions and tomatoes. Other phytochemicals are unique to particular plants, such as allicin in garlic and onions, which can fight infections and help reduce the risk of developing some cancers, piperine in pepper, which can reduce blood pressure and inflammation and thymoquinone in black cumin, which can boost immunity.

Some wild plants, especially Australian native plants, have high concentrations of phytochemicals. Kakadu plums (*Terminalia ferdinandiana*) have some of the highest recorded concentrations of vitamin C, plus other beneficial phytochemicals, such as ellagic and gallic acids. Davidsonia plums (*Davidsonia pruriens*) contain phytochemicals with antioxidant and anti-inflammatory potentials greater than blueberries (Sakulnarmrat 2012). The wild herb gotu kola (*Centella asiatica*) has been found to improve mental performance and mood in some people (Wattanathorn *et al.*

2008). Wild fruits also typically contain higher amounts of fibre than cultivated fruits (Brand-Miller & Holt 1998).

Many phytochemicals provide health benefits through the same actions as some medicinal drugs. For example, aspirin is a medicine originally derived from the phytochemical salicylic acid, concentrated in the bark of willow trees (*Salix* species) and the herb meadowsweet (*Filipendula ulmaria*). Aspirin reduces pain and inflammation, and thins the blood, by inhibiting an enzyme in our cells that leads to inflammation. Enzymes are proteins that speed up chemical reactions in our bodies. Many phytochemicals, such as those in ginger and olives, provide similar benefits to aspirin by inhibiting the same enzyme. While phytochemicals in edible plants may not be consumed or absorbed at the same concentration as drugs, and therefore not provide symptom relief as rapidly as drugs, they typically have no side effects and often provide multiple benefits throughout our bodies.

In addition to phytochemicals, fruit, vegetables, herbs and spices provide abundant proteins, minerals and fibre. While proteins, minerals and fibre are not the focus of this book, a regular supply of each is clearly essential. In fact, many people may be deficient in some minerals and trace elements, such as magnesium, selenium and zinc, and this may contribute to some chronic diseases like depression and high blood pressure (Hungerford 2012). A diet with a wide variety of fresh fruit, vegetables, herbs and spices can usually supply adequate quantities of minerals, although some people may find particular supplements helpful.

In his 2015 book, *The Dorito Effect*, Mark Shatzker argued that our taste receptors are programmed to seek out chemicals that are associated with important nutrients. For example, the aromatic chemicals that we link with flavour in tomatoes are associated with essential nutrients (Goff & Klee 2006).

Artificial flavours mimic the taste of many phytochemicals and cater to our craving for them. There is no better evidence of our desire for phytochemicals than the staggering efforts people went to in the pursuit of spices. The principal spices, nutmeg, pepper, cloves, cinnamon, ginger and turmeric originate from Asia, especially India and Indonesia. These spices have been traded through Asia and the Middle East for thousands of years and propelled the expansion of European empires from the late 15th century. While certainly helping to flavour food, there is evidence that spices were also sought after for their medicinal properties.

The zeal and wealth provided by the trade in spices is difficult to comprehend today, given our ease of access to them. Pepper, for example, was a spice of the wealthy. It was demanded, along with gold and silver, as a ransom payment in the fifth century AD by Alaric the Visigoth, to abandon his siege of Rome.

The development of artificial flavouring is an enormous modern industry, reflecting our desire for the spicy tastes provided by phytochemicals. Given that some fruit and vegetables seem to have become increasingly bland in recent decades, it is probably no surprise that there is evidence the nutritional concentration of some cultivated fruit and vegetables has declined in the last 50 to 70 years (Davis 2009). Organic produce is thought by some people to be more nutritious and tasty than conventionally grown food (i.e. using artificial fertilisers and pesticides). There have been mixed reports from studies on whether organic or conventionally-grown produce has a greater concentration of minerals. However, plants that must deal with insect attack and are not pampered with excessive fertiliser (e.g. organically grown plants) typically have a higher phytochemical concentration (Barański et al. 2014; Heimler et al. 2017). This is no surprise, because many phytochemicals are made by plants in response to insect herbivory and to allow them to grow in conditions they would experience in the wild. For example, tomatoes grown organically have been found to have higher levels of two health-providing flavonoids, kaempferol and quercetin, than conventionally grown tomatoes (Mitchell *et al.* 2007).

Consistently, nutritional recommendations advise that we should eat a large amount of fresh fruit and vegetables daily. The World Cancer Research Fund International recommends eating at least five servings (totalling about 400 grams) of a variety of non-starchy vegetables and fruit every day to reduce the risk of cancer. Similarly, Australian dietary guidelines recommend two serves of fruit and five to six serves of vegetables each day. This is a fair amount of fruit and vegetables, and most Australians are not eating anywhere near this quantity (Hendrie & Noakes 2017). There is related advice to eat a kaleidoscope of colourful fruit and vegetables to provide a diversity of phytochemicals. The reasons why eating a variety of fresh fruit, vegetables, herbs and spices benefit our health are the subject of this book.

Plants are great for our health because they provide direct antioxidant actions, as well as stimulating our cells to make our own antioxidants. Amazingly, some phytochemicals activate a protein within our cells that copies genetic information from our DNA to make powerful antioxidants. This is an astonishing discovery: that phytochemicals in plants such as blueberries, broccoli, garlic and turmeric, influence how our bodies use our genetic information. Phytochemicals also enhance our body's ability to reduce inflammation and can inhibit the growth of tumours. For example ellagic acid, found in several fruit such as strawberries, can reduce the growth of new blood vessels around tumours (Labrecque *et al.* 2005).

Different phytochemicals complement each other, and this explains the need for eating a wide variety of plants. In one study, eating whole tomatoes reduced prostate tumour size in laboratory rats to a greater extent than purified lycopene (a phytochemical in tomatoes), and the combination of tomatoes and broccoli reduced tumour size to a greater extent than just tomatoes or broccoli individually (Canene-Adams *et al.* 2007).

As a result of their antioxidant, anti-inflammatory and other actions, phytochemicals can help lower the risk of developing cardiovascular disease, type 2 diabetes, dementia and some cancers. This book provides a review of phytochemicals and why plants make them. Summary information is given for common fruit, vegetables, herbs and spices and plant products such as tea and dark chocolate. Additional information is presented on the phytochemicals of some Australian native bush food plants, which are rightly attracting increased nutritional attention.

Chapter 2
Overview of phytochemicals

Although in the broad sense, phytochemicals cover all chemicals produced by plants, the term is used throughout this book to focus on secondary metabolites, which are chemicals made by plants that are not primary nutrients. That is, this book concentrates on phytochemicals that are not sugars, proteins and fats. Phytochemicals are the colourful pigments in fruit, the flavour of spices and the stimulants in coffee and tea. We consume abundant phytochemicals in coffee, dark chocolate, tea and wine.

Morphine was the first phytochemical isolated in a laboratory. This chemical achievement was performed by Friedrich Sertürner, who extracted morphine from opium poppies in 1806 (Atanasov *et al.* 2015). Sertürner initially tested the effect of morphine on a dog and then, in the time-honoured way of scientists, he tested it on himself. He named the compound after the Greek god of dreams, Morpheus, which provides a hint about the effect it had on him. Soon after Sertürner's extraction of morphine, many other phytochemicals were isolated from plants, including caffeine, cocaine, codeine and quinine.

Gradually over time, thousands of phytochemicals have been detected. Phytochemicals are typically grouped into broad categories, such as those shown in Figure 2.1 and Tables 2.1 and 2.2, on the basis of their chemical structures. Greater detail about each phytochemical group is provided in Chapter 13 and why plants make them in the first place, in Chapter 14.

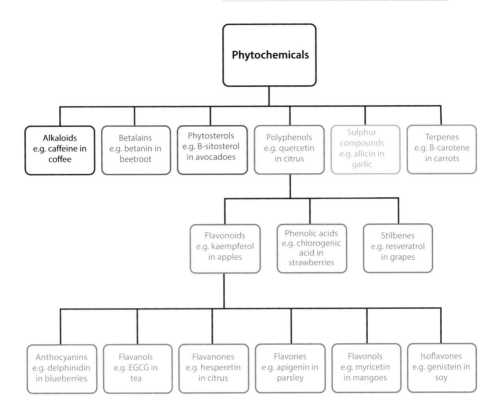

Figure 2.1. Broad groups of phytochemicals that provide health benefits, and examples of plants in which they are found. The polyphenols have a diverse range of health-promoting phytochemicals and subgroups are shown. For example, delphinidin, a type of anthocyanin found in blueberries, (bottom left) is an example of a flavonoid. Flavonoids are a subset of polyphenols, which are one of six broad categories of phytochemicals. Note that most vitamins can also be considered phytochemicals.

Table 2.1. Summary of the broad groups of phytochemicals and their key health benefits

Phytochemical group	Characteristics and examples	Example plants containing them	Key potential health benefits
Alkaloids	Contain nitrogen, e.g. capsaicin, caffeine and theobromine	Capsicums, coffee, tea and dark chocolate	Stimulants, capsaicin may reduce pain perception
Betalains	Also contain nitrogen, e.g. betanin and indicaxanthin.	Beetroots, prickly pear cactus and dragon fruit	Antioxidants, reduce inflammatory pain, increase nitric oxide-stimulated blood flow
Phytosterols	Have a similar chemical structure to cholesterol, e.g. beta-sitosterol and campesterol	Legumes, whole grains, avocados and some nuts (e.g. macadamias)	Can balance cholesterol improving heart health, potentially contribute to lowering cancer risk
Polyphenols	Based on a central six carbon ring, include resveratrol, curcumin, gingerol and flavonoids, e.g. quercetin	Very abundant in fruit, vegetables, herbs and spices, including citrus, ginger, grapes and turmeric	Antioxidant, anti-inflammatory, lower allergy symptoms, improve cardiovascular health and help inhibit cancer development

Table 2.1. *continued...*

Phytochemical group	Characteristics and examples	Example plants containing them	Key potential health benefits
Sulphur compounds	Contain sulphur, e.g. allicin and sulforaphane	Garlic, broccoli, cabbage, kale and onions	Antioxidants, reduce inflammation, help inhibit cancer development, thin the blood and maintain healthy blood vessels
Terpenes	Fat soluble, provide yellow to red colours, e.g. beta-carotene, lutein and lycopene	Carrots, spinach and tomatoes	Anti-cancer properties, essential for eye health, some are a precursor to vitamin A

Polyphenols are a large group of health-stimulating phyto-chemicals. They include flavonoids, phenolic acids and stil-benes. Many phenolic acids, such as caffeic acid in blueberries and coffee, have only a single phenol, rather than multiple or *poly-phenols*. Other phenolic acids, such as ellagic acid in peaches and strawberries, contain multiple phenols. Flavonoids, sometimes called bioflavonoids or vitamin P, are a significant group of polyphenols. Common flavonoids consumed include apigenin (in celery and parsley), delphinidin (from blueberries and wine), hesperetin (in oranges and mandarins), kaemp-ferol (in apples and tea), myricetin (in mangoes, coffee and tea), naringenin (in grapefruit and oranges) and quercetin (via apples, grapes, broccoli, onions and tea; Somerset & Johannot 2008). Several types of flavonoids differ in chemical structure and effect, providing subgroups.

Table 2.2. Summary of flavonoid subgroups (all of which are polyphenols)

Flavonoid group	Example phytochemicals	Example plants	Key potential health benefits
Anthocyanins	Delphinidin	Blueberries	Contribute antioxidant, anti-inflammatory, anti-cancer and brain function boosting effects
Flavanols	Catechins and theaflavins	Tea	Increase the antioxidant capacity in blood, reduce inflammation and oxidation of LDL 'bad' cholesterol
Flavanones	Hesperetin and naringenin	Citrus	Can help lessen allergic responses by reducing histamine production, may enhance vitamin C benefits
Flavones	Apigenin and luteolin	Celery, parsley and lemon grass	Can reduce oxidation of LDL 'bad' cholesterol
Flavonols	Kaempferol, myricetin and quercetin	Apples, capsicums, onions, oranges, strawberries, tomatoes	Can help reduce allergy symptoms, inflammation and oxidation of LDLs
Isoflavones	Genistein and daidzein	Legumes such as lentils and soybeans	Help balance cholesterol and may lower breast and prostate cancer risk

Chapter 3

Eating plants, and their phytochemicals, contributes to long-term good health

The Australian dietary guidelines recommend adults eat two serves of fruit and five to six serves of vegetables each day. An example of this would be eating an apple and an orange, a cup of cooked vegetables and four cups of salad vegetables daily. Consuming this quantity of fruit and vegetables requires plants to dominate most meals. Recent studies indicate the majority of Australians are not meeting the recommended target, with obese Australians eating the least fruit and vegetables (Hendrie & Noakes 2017).

Other countries, such as Canada, France, New Zealand, UK and USA, have similar dietary guidelines to eat plenty of fruit and vegetables. Various national guidelines also encourage eating a wide range of different plants providing a broad spectrum of colours.

Why is there a consistent push to eat so many fruit and vegetables and what is the basis of this advice? Studies that look at the pattern of diseases with diet and lifestyle (called epidemiology) consistently link a high intake of fruit and vegetables with long-term health. Of course, associating disease with diet only identifies patterns and there may be confounding factors contributing to the health effects. For example, people eating a lot of fruit and vegetables may also undertake a lot of exercise, and exercise may be contributing to the health benefits observed. In recent decades an understanding of precisely how plant foods provide their array of health benefits has been building, through the combination of laboratory studies examining the response of human cells to phytochemicals in Petri dishes and test tubes, animal studies looking at different food and compounds on specific diseases, and human trials. Each of these methods: epidemiology studies, laboratory experiments, animal studies and human trials, contribute unique evidence to the broader picture, although each type of study has its own limitations. The combined results of these studies show many phytochemicals, obtained by eating a variety of fruit, vegetables, herbs and spices, are essential elements of long-term, good health. A summary of the key evidence is provided in this and the following chapters.

People living in communities that are renowned for longevity and a healthy old age (so called blue zones) typically consume large amounts of fruit and vegetables (Buettner 2015). For example, people on the Greek island of Ikaria include over 150 wild vegetables and herbs in their diet, while elders on the Japanese islands of Okinawa also eat a plant-rich diet. Although the specific diets of various blue zones differ, and the role of community involvement and regular exercise is central, a universal element is their plant-rich eating habits.

Studies that follow large numbers of people over many decades provide valuable information. A recent review of several studies following a total of 833,234 people for between five and 26 years found clear benefits in the consumption of fruit and vegetables in reducing mortality rates, especially from cardiovascular disease (Wang *et al.* 2014). A forty year Norwegian study of about 10,000 men found those who ate the most fruit and vegetables delayed their risk of death from cancer and stroke, meaning they were healthy for longer (Hjartåker *et al.* 2015). The North American Nurses' Study, established in 1976 and involving over 280,000 people, has provided exceptional information on diet and lifestyle.

A complementary Health Professionals Follow-Up Study has tracked the health of over 50,000 men since 1986. These long term studies have linked the consumption of fruit and vegetables with lower rates of various diseases including type 2 diabetes (Korat *et al.* 2014), cardiovascular disease (Yu *et al.* 2016) and Parkinson's disease (Gao *et al.* 2012). Herb and spice consumption is also linked with health benefits. For example, Brits of Indian ancestry who eat a lot of spices such as turmeric, tend to have a lower incidence of cancer than others in the UK (Ali *et al.* 2010).

Intervention trials which look at changes in people once they increase their fruit and vegetable intake provide further evidence. American doctor, Dean Ornish, has documented dramatic improvements in cardiovascular health, including some reversal of blood vessel blockages, in people who have changed their lifestyle by eating a vegetarian diet low in fat, coupled with exercise, group support and meditation (Ornish *et al.* 1990; 1998; Ornish & Ornish 2019).

In the 1970s, people in North Karalia, a region in northern Finland, reduced the rate of lung cancer in middle aged men by 10% and of heart attacks by 25%, by decreasing the number of smokers (from around half to a third of men), reducing animal fats and increasing vegetables in their diet (Buettner 2015). In her comprehensively researched book, *Death by Food Pyramid*, Denise Minger (2013) pointed out that three of the current popular eating patterns that have evidence of health benefits (Paleo-Primal, Mediterranean, and Whole foods plant-based diets) have significant differences, but the three eating styles overlap in minimising processed food and including considerable quantities of low sugar fruit and non-starchy vegetables.

Given the evidence that eating fruit, vegetables, herbs and spices is important for maintaining and even restoring health, the obvious question is why. Why is it healthy to eat a lot of plants? To understand this, we need to consider how our bodies function.

Our bodies operate through the process of metabolism, which is the combination of activities in our cells that create energy, growth and healing. This occurs through step-wise chemical reactions, described as metabolic pathways. These pathways are extremely complex yet occur continuously, at lightning speed within our cells. This complex efficiency is the beauty of biochemistry.

Phytochemicals can play a part in various stages of these metabolic pathways. They can contribute directly, or indirectly by promoting enzymes that catalyse chemical reactions and stimulating cell responses to mild stress (Ong *et al.* 2017).

Phytochemicals influence how the information in our genes is used. Genes are the basis of our family characteristics. They are segments of our DNA that our cells use as a recipe to produce proteins that drive our metabolism. We are born with a specific genetic blueprint, but our health is not an inevitable consequence of our genes. Genes are turned on and off by elements of our lifestyle, including diet, exercise and exposure to toxins. Amazingly, many phytochemicals stimulate proteins called transcription factors within our cells, which cause the translation of genetic information in DNA to make compounds essential to our wellbeing. For example, many phytochemicals trigger a transcription factor called Nrf2 to transcribe genetic information to produce antioxidant compounds.

Recent progress in determining people's genetic makeup has led to speculations that some variants of certain genes are associated with specific diseases. One example is the gene that codes for the protein apolipoprotein E (ApoE). Apolipoprotein mixes with fats to form lipoproteins that carry fats and cholesterol in the blood (e.g. low density lipoproteins, LDLs). There are several variations of the ApoE gene, and the variant called ApoE4 has been found to be associated with a higher incidence of some chronic diseases such as Alzheimer's disease and atherosclerosis (cardiovascular disease). Compared to other ApoE variants, people with ApoE4 tend to have a higher level of cholesterol in their blood and ApoE4 is associated with increased inflammation in the brain. However, a diet that reduces chronic inflammation and maintains a healthy cholesterol level can help override a genetic predisposition.

A small amount of stress from exercise or brief fasting is good for us. Exercising encourages our muscles and cardiovascular system to respond to the stress of weights or exertion by growing muscle and improving circulation. Short-term calorie restriction (i.e. fasting) is thought to be a stress that slows ageing through a variety of processes, such as promoting antioxidants, reducing inflammation and increasing insulin sensitivity (Van Cauwenberghe *et al.* 2016; Teruya *et al.* 2019). Calorie restriction also promotes cell maintenance by lowering the levels of a protein called mTOR, while increasing another protein called AMPK (DiNicolantonio & Fung 2019).

Providing mild metabolic stress is thought to be one of the ways some phytochemicals are good for us. Some of these mild stress-promoting phytochemicals are produced by plants to repel or even kill bacteria, fungi, insects and other herbivores. These plant toxins are consumed at low doses when we eat healthy amounts of fruit, vegetables, herbs and spices. Our cells respond by making antioxidants and other beneficial compounds to reduce the stress and in the process build a healthier cell (Surh 2011; Menendez *et al.* 2013). For example, the phytochemical resveratrol, which protects grapes from fungal attack (Jeandet *et al.* 2014), promotes antioxidants and activates a beneficial protein called sirtuin 1. Several phytochemicals can also lower mTOR levels and increase AMPK. These include phytochemicals in garlic, grapes, green tea, olives and turmeric (Pallauf *et al.* 2013; Willcox & Willcox 2014; DiNicolantonio & Fung 2019).

In summary, phytochemicals can provide health benefits by acting as direct antioxidants, and by promoting our cells to make our own antioxidants. They can reduce chronic inflammation, inhibit the formation of new blood vessels around tumours and fat tissue, and help with reducing weight. As a result, phytochemicals can contribute to reducing the risk of developing, or the severity of, various conditions such as cardiovascular disease, some cancers and type 2 diabetes. These beneficial actions of phytochemicals are discussed in the next chapters.

Chapter 4
Phytochemicals provide antioxidant benefits

The direct antioxidant properties of phytochemicals

KEY POINTS

- Our cells are exposed to oxidation from free radicals every day and the resulting damage contributes to diseases such as dementia, cardiovascular disease and some cancers.
- Phytochemicals provide direct antioxidant benefits by stabilising free radicals.
- Examples of the many plants providing antioxidant phytochemicals include apples, blueberries, carrots, cabbage family vegetables, citrus, garlic, ginger, grapes, onions, oregano, pomegranate, rosemary, tea and turmeric.

The word antioxidant pops up regularly in discussions about the health benefits of fruit and vegetables. Antioxidants are important for stopping the oxidising damage to our bodies caused by compounds called free radicals. Oxidation is a chemistry term describing the loss, or sharing, of one or more electrons (negatively charged particles) from an atom or molecule. This often occurs when oxygen is joined to a molecule (therefore is called 'oxidation') or a hydrogen atom is removed. The browning of a sliced apple and the rusting of iron are examples of oxidation. In both cases there has been a chemical change, and when this occurs in our bodies it can cause ageing and contribute to a range of chronic diseases, including heart disease.

The term 'free radical' refers to a molecule within or around our cells that is unstable as a result of an unpaired electron. These free radicals are then compelled to steal an electron from another molecule, causing oxidative damage to proteins, DNA and fats. Antioxidants have the useful ability to give up an electron to free radicals, while resisting the temptation to steal an electron from another molecule. That is, the domino effect of electron thieving and damage stops with antioxidants. Plants make various phytochemicals to work as antioxidants to protect themselves from free radicals (discussed further in Chapter 14). We receive the benefits of plant antioxidants when we eat fruit, vegetables, herbs and spices.

Free radicals are formed continuously within our bodies. For example, free radicals are created as an inadvertent side-effect of energy production within mitochondria (the tiny energy producing units in our cells). Healthy mitochondria produce energy while emitting only low levels of free radicals, while damaged mitochondria release more free radicals from the imperfect combustion of glucose with oxygen. Free radicals can also develop following exposure to radiation, some chemicals (e.g. cigarette smoke) and UV light.

A low level of free radicals in the right place is beneficial. Our immune system employs the toxic nature of free radicals to destroy disease-causing microbes. However, when out of balance or in the wrong location, free radicals are thought to contribute to a range of diseases, including inflammation, athero-sclerosis and therefore heart disease, Alzheimer's disease, and lung and liver cancer (Di Meo *et al.* 2013). An extreme example of the damage from free radicals is radiation poisoning, in which excessive oxidation overwhelms our organs.

Free radicals are thought to contribute to heart disease, for example, by oxidising the fats and cholesterol transported through our blood vessels within low density lipoproteins (the

LDLs discussed by doctors in relation to 'bad' cholesterol). Our blood is water-based and as fat does not dissolve in water, fats and cholesterol are transported through our blood within packets called lipoproteins. Lipoproteins range in size from very low density, to low density and high density (HDL). LDLs can be further divided into whether they are large and fluffy or relatively small and dense. The small and dense LDLs, promoted with the consumption of sugar and other refined carbohydrates (Hyman 2016), are considered more dangerous and are most likely to be oxidised (Brukner 2018). Unfortunately most research reports, and many blood tests, do not distinguish between these two types of LDLs.

LDLs carry fats and cholesterol to cells and their overabundance is considered by many to be an important indicator of cardiovascular disease. Excess LDLs can remain circulating within the blood and become damaged by oxidation. HDLs clean up fats and cholesterol in the blood and return them to the liver, which is why it is considered good to have ample HDLs in proportion to LDLs. Therefore many people think that it is not just the amount of LDLs, but the ratio of HDLs to LDLs and whether LDLs have been damaged by free radical oxidation, which contributes to atherosclerosis and associated heart disease and stroke (Lobo *et al.* 2010; Gillespie 2013).

The more fruit and vegetables eaten on a regular basis, the lower the levels of oxidation damage, including of LDL 'bad' cholesterol and DNA (Pedret *et al.* 2012; Cocate *et al.* 2014). Drinking a strawberry drink containing the equivalent of 110 grams of strawberries has been found to reduce the oxidation damage to LDLs after people ate a high fat meal (Burton-Freeman *et al.* 2010). Vitamin E and other phytochemicals, such as those found in grapes and minimally processed dark chocolate called procyanidins, and beta-carotene in carrots, also reduce the oxidation of LDL 'bad' cholesterol in blood vessels (Elliott & Elliott 2009).

Vitamin C in fruit and vegetables is a powerful antioxidant. Interestingly, the vitamin C within an apple provides only a small proportion of the apple's overall antioxidant capacity (Eberhardt *et al.* 2000). The combination of many phyto-chemicals in an apple, working synergistically, produces its full antioxidant potential (Liu 2003).

The antioxidant capacity of different plants can be estimated in the laboratory using chemical tests. These assessments are not perfect, but give an indication of relative antioxidant potential. A standard test that rates the degree to which fruit, vegetables, herbs and spices inhibit oxidation in a laboratory setting is described in ORAC units (oxygen radical absorbance capacity; Haytowitz & Bhagwat 2010). Another antioxidant scale is FRAP (ferric-ion reducing antioxidant power). Herbs and spices typically have considerably higher ORAC scores than fruit and vegetables. For example, the ORAC scores of dried oregano (175,295), dried rosemary (165,280) and ground turmeric (127,068) are dramatically higher than red apples (4,275), oranges (2,103) and iceberg lettuce (438; Haytowitz & Bhagwat 2010). However, it is important to note that these ORAC scores are based on 100 grams of produce, and it would require many meals to consume 100 grams of herbs and spices, whereas we can easily consume several hundred grams of fruit and vegetables each day.

Eating a range of plants provides a diversity of phytochemi-cals with antioxidant properties. Some phytochemicals are fat soluble and are therefore better absorbed when eaten with fats, such as olive oil. Because they mix with fats, they are particu-larly important for helping protect fat-transporting LDLs from oxidative damage that can lead to atherosclerosis. Examples of fat soluble phytochemicals are vitamin E and beta-carotene in carrots, which is a pre-curser from which our bodies can make vitamin A. Lycopene, which provides the red colouring of tomatoes and red grapefruit and has been shown to help fight cancer development, is another fat-soluble antioxidant. Lutein and zeaxanthin, which are fat soluble carotenoids found in dark leafy vegetables, corn, oranges and Kiwi fruit, are actively absorbed into the retina of our eyes, where they provide essential protection against the oxidation damage that can cause macular degeneration and cataracts.

Phytochemicals that are water soluble include flavonoids, such as anthocyanins in blueberries and catechins in tea. The antioxidant capacity of flavonoids contributes to their many benefits, such as reducing oxidative damage to blood vessels and brain cells.

Phytochemicals stimulate our bodies to generate antioxidants

> ### KEY POINTS
>
> - Phytochemicals amplify the antioxidant capacity of our cells.
> - They achieve this by activating a protein within our cells called Nrf2, which increases the production of powerful antioxidants, especially glutathione.
> - There are many plants with phytochemicals that do this, including allicin in garlic, anthocyanins in blueberries, apigenin in parsley, curcumin in turmeric, hydroxytyrosol in olives, lycopene in tomatoes, quercetin in citrus and onions, sulforaphane in broccoli and cabbages plus catechins and theaflavins in tea.

The direct antioxidant properties of phytochemicals are just one aspect of the health benefits plants provide. Numerous human studies demonstrate a significant increase in the antioxidant capacity of blood plasma after eating fruit and vegetables. However, the increased antioxidant activity is typically much greater than can be accounted for by the small rise in plasma concentrations of phytochemicals (Lotito & Frei 2006). It is apparent that phytochemicals are crucial in amplifying the antioxidant capacity of our cells.

The direct antioxidant effects of phytochemicals are particularly valuable to our digestive tract, and are linked to lower rates of throat, stomach and colon cancer. However, a proportion of phytochemicals can pass straight through our digestive system. Some phytochemicals that enter our blood stream have been chemically changed in the stomach, intestines and liver by enzymes and gut bacteria. These changes often involve simply removing a sugar molecule attached to the phytochemical or splitting the phytochemical into smaller compounds. Therefore, phytochemicals that are absorbed from the intestines into the blood stream can be an altered, though still effective, version of the molecule that we have eaten (Del Rio *et al.* 2013).

At the concentrations that reach the cells across our body, phytochemicals probably only directly affect a relatively small concentration of free radicals. In the process of quenching a free radical, the phytochemicals are altered themselves into a free radical-like state called an electrophile (Forman *et al.* 2014). Even at low concentrations, the phytochemicals in an electrophile state provide a very significant indirect antioxidant role by stimulating our cells to make powerful antioxidants, especially glutathione and superoxide dismutase (SOD). This is probably the most valuable antioxidant benefit that phytochemicals provide, and echoes some of their actions within plants themselves.

Phytochemicals stimulate our cells to manufacture antioxidants by activating a protein called Nrf2, a type of transcription factor, which builds compounds from genetic recipes stored in

DNA. As mentioned earlier, the activation of Nrf2 causes the reading of genetic information in our DNA, stimulating our cells to make highly efficient antioxidants, such as SOD and glutathione (Li *et al.* 2016). Evidence is accumulating that a wide range of phytochemicals can activate the protein Nrf2 and its related benefits. These include curcumin from turmeric, epigallocatechin-3-gallate in green tea, polyphenols in olive oil, quercetin in citrus, onions and tomatoes, resveratrol in grapes, sulforaphane in plants of the cabbage family, terpenoids found in basil, cranberries, grapefruit and many other plants, and allicin from garlic and onions (Surh 2011; Menendez *et al.* 2013).

One small trial provided a simple demonstration of the role of phytochemicals in stimulating our cells to make antioxidants. Fourteen participants initially ate a diet very low in flavonoids and other natural antioxidants for a week, leading to a decrease in glutathione reductase (which activates glutathione) and SOD concentrations within their red blood cells (Nielsen *et al.* 1999). These low levels were associated with increased oxidative damage to proteins in their blood. Levels of glutathione reductase and SOD increased again within red blood cells once people started eating parsley, which provided the flavonoid apigenin.

In another study, 18 people who drank berry juice high in polyphenols, increased their glutathione levels and reduced the amount of oxidised LDL 'bad' cholesterol (Weisel *et al.* 2006). This stimulation of the powerful antioxidant glutathione was not observed in nine participants who drank a placebo lacking polyphenols.

Eating a variety of fruit, vegetables, herbs and spices provides complementary benefits. For example, several carotenoids found in tomatoes work together in combination to reduce prostate cell growth in laboratory tests to a greater extent than just the carotenoid lycopene alone (Linnewiel-Hermoni *et al.* 2015). The activation of the protein Nrf2 by many phytochemicals, such as epigallocatechin-3-gallate in green tea, causes a succession of health benefits by promoting glutathione production. Glutathione is a powerful antioxidant by itself and complements vitamin E in inhibiting the oxidation of fats and therefore protecting against cardiovascular disease. Glutathione combines with the carotenoids lutein and zeaxanthin in providing antioxidant benefits that protect our eyes from oxidative damage that leads to cataracts and macular degeneration. Glutathione also recharges the antioxidant capacity of vitamin C, so that each vitamin C molecule can stabilise multiple free radicals (Leong & Ko 2016).

Interestingly, there is emerging evidence that not only does too little Nrf2 increase our cells' susceptibility to carcinogens, oxidative damage and infections, but that a rapid activation of too much Nrf2 (especially in response to strong toxins, such as arsenic) is linked to drug resistance and cancer cell proliferation (Huang *et al.* 2015). This suggests that the constant low-level bioavailability of Nrf2-stimulating phytochemicals, such as sulforaphane from broccoli and curcuminoids from turmeric, provide beneficial Nrf2 concentrations; but powerful toxins, like arsenic, activate too much Nrf2 too quickly, causing cell damage.

In summary, phytochemicals supplied by a wide range of plants reduce oxidative damage to cells and tissues, including of blood vessels and brain cells. Phytochemicals provide significant health benefits through their capacity as direct antioxidants and also through their ability to stimulate our cells to make powerful antioxidants such as glutathione (Figure 4.1). Combined, this antioxidant function reduces corrosion from free radicals. In doing so, these antioxidants help protect against a range of diseases, including cardiovascular disease, some cancers and dementia.

Some phytochemicals, such as beta-carotene in carrots and lycopene in tomatoes, are fat soluble and are best absorbed when eaten with fats, such as olive oil. They are important for helping protect cholesterol and fat transporting LDLs from oxidative damage, therefore help protect against atherosclerosis. Water-soluble phytochemicals include flavonoids such as anthocyanins in blueberries and catechins in tea. The antioxidant capacity of these water-soluble flavonoids helps reduce oxidative damage to blood vessels and brain cells.

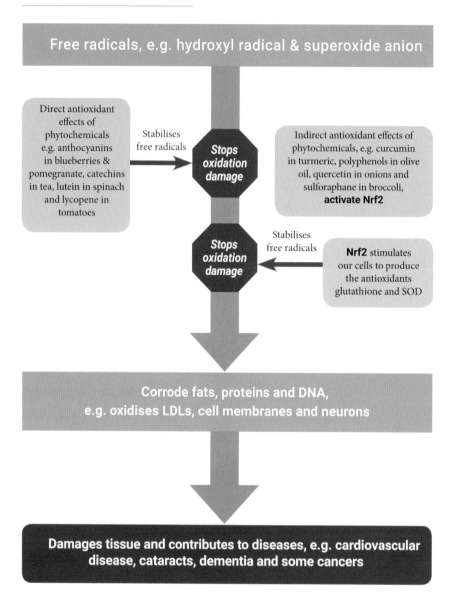

Figure 4.1. Diagrammatic representation of the direct and indirect antioxidant functions of phytochemicals that stabilise free radicals, inhibiting their damage and helping reduce the risk of developing several diseases.

Chapter 5

Phytochemicals help reduce chronic inflammation

KEY POINTS

- Inflammation is necessary for healing wounds and infections. It can also occur following oxidation damage to cells from free radicals. When inflammation does not switch off, it causes significant damage to tissues, contributing to diseases such as arthritis, cardiovascular disease, dementia and some cancers.

- Phytochemicals relieve chronic inflammation by inhibiting proteins that make inflammatory compounds. They complement omega 3 fats, such as ALA in flax seed and purslane, which our bodies use to make anti-inflammatory compounds.

- Phytochemicals that help reduce inflammation include anthocyanins in blueberries and cherries, capsaicin in capsicum and chillies, carnosol in rosemary and sage, catechins in tea, curcumin in turmeric, diallyl disulfide in garlic, eugenol in cloves, gingerol in ginger, kaempferol in apples, piperine in pepper, quercetin in citrus and onions, resveratrol in grapes and sulforaphane in broccoli, Brussels sprouts and cabbages.

Inflammation is the painful red swelling we experience after an injury. When we cut our skin or have a bacterial infection, part of our immune response is to create inflammation. This achieves several useful outcomes, including killing pathogens with free radicals, dismantling and removing injured cells, establishing a good blood supply to help healing and sending a message to the brain, interpreted as pain, to limit movement of an injured limb. Unfortunately, inflammatory compounds that attack bacteria and dissolve injured cells, can also damage adjacent healthy tissue if the inflammation is not resolved.

In response to an injury, infection or cell death, white blood cells (which are immune cells in our blood and lymphatic system) release compounds that cause a cascade of events leading to inflammation. Specifically, white blood cells secrete compounds called chemokines and cytokines that send a message to local cells, or travel through our blood to communicate with distant cells, to activate inflammation. These messenger compounds cause the activation of a protein known as NF-κB. Tobacco smoke, free radicals and high blood glucose levels may also activate NF-κB (Anand *et al.* 2008; Morgan *et al.* 2011; Nareika *et al.* 2008). NF-kB is a transcription factor that triggers genetic information in our DNA to be used to produce compounds that promote inflammation. NF-kB causes the production of the enzyme cyclooxygenase 2 (COX-2), which catalyses the manufacture of the inflammatory compound prostaglandin E2 from omega 6 fats (Elliott & Elliott 2009; Lim *et al.* 2001). The resulting inflammation includes the stimulation of nerve receptors to transmit the perception of pain.

Once a wound has healed, or an infection is remedied, our bodies have a process to actively end inflammation. This involves several compounds with appropriate names such as resolvins and protectins, which are made from omega 3 fats (found for example in fish and flax seed). Resolvins inhibit the production of further inflammatory compounds and promote anti-inflammatory compounds such as a cytokine called interleukin-10 (Lim *et al.* 2015). Protectins help turn off inflammation in the brain. If the inflammation is not ended through this process, or there is constant irritation or high levels of inflammation promoting molecules present in our circulation, then the inflammation persists.

When the inflammation does not turn off, it is called chronic inflammation. The immune system starts to attack healthy tissue, such as brain cells and blood vessels, or overreacts to harmless proteins, triggering allergies. The tissue damage caused by ongoing inflammation is a significant health issue, thought to contribute to many diseases, including autoimmune diseases, dementia, heart disease and strokes (via atherosclerosis in blood vessels) and some cancers (Rock & Kono 2008; Devi *et al.* 2015). Unresolved inflammation contributes to the pain and swelling associated with arthritis. It also triggers the release of histamines that, when inappropriate, cause allergic reactions.

Eating plenty of plants can help reduce inflammation and allergies. For example, a survey of 690 children in Crete found those who regularly ate fruit such as apples, grapes, oranges and tomatoes, had lower incidents of hay fever and asthma-like symptoms such as wheezing (Chatzi *et al.* 2007).

A diet containing an overabundance of seed oils (most vegetable oils) high in omega 6 fats (especially from refined corn, cotton, soybeans and sunflower seeds) can contribute to chronic inflammation, because these fats are the building material for inflammatory compounds (Patterson *et al.* 2012). Many of these oils are used in processed foods. Omega 6 fats are named because their molecule has a double bond between carbon atoms at the sixth carbon from the end (omega being the last letter of the Greek alphabet). The omega 6 fat, linoleic acid, is converted to arachidonic acid, which the enzyme COX-2 uses to manufacture the inflammatory compound prostaglandin E2. Arachidonic acid can also be used by the enzyme 5-lipoxygenase (5-LOX) to make other inflammatory compounds called leukotrienes.

Omega 6 fats
e.g. linoleic acid in corn, cotton, soy and sunflower seed oils

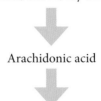

Arachidonic acid

Inflammatory compounds
e.g. prostaglandin E2 and leukotrienes

In contrast to omega 6 fats, our bodies use omega 3 fats to make anti-inflammatory compounds, such as prostaglandin E1, resolvins and protectins. Omega 3 fats include alpha-linolenic acid (ALA) which is produced by plants, especially in chloroplasts within leaves where photosynthesis occurs. It is abundant in flax seed, purslane, spinach and watercress (Pereira *et al.* 2001). Eicosapentaenoic acid (EPA) and docosahexaenoic acid (DHA) from fish, especially wild salmon and sardines (with smaller concentrations in pasture-fed livestock) are other types of omega 3 fats. They play important roles throughout our body, including making our cell membranes more flexible and EPA is important for reducing excessive blood clotting.

Our brains and eyes require the DHA form of omega 3. Only a small proportion of the plant-sourced ALA that we eat is converted in our bodies to EPA then onto DHA; although eating plenty of plants will ensure there is abundant ALA to contribute to the process. This is less efficient than simply eating DHA in fish. However, good wild sources of fish are becoming more difficult to keep sustainable, and farmed fish sometimes contain lower levels of DHA than wild fish (though still at valuable levels), depending on what they are fed.

Studies indicate vegans (who do not acquire DHA directly from fish, meat or eggs), especially male vegans, typically have lower levels of DHA in their blood than meat and fish eaters (Rosell *et al*. 2005; Welsh *et al*. 2010). However, fish obtain their DHA from microalgae, and microalgae oil may be another option for sourcing DHA (Doughman *et al*. 2007). There is also some evidence from rodent studies that the brain may conserve DHA, meaning the differences in long term DHA levels stored in the brain may be relatively minimal, irrespective of whether it was obtained directly from fish etc. or by converting ALA from plants (Domenichiello *et al*. 2015). The conversion of plant-sourced omega 3 ALA to DHA in our bodies is reduced when we eat a lot of the omega 6 linoleic acid, because they compete for a common enzyme used in their metabolism. Therefore it would be wise to not consume excessive amounts of omega 6 fats, especially from highly processed products. The combination of turmeric with pepper, may help the conversion of ALA consumed in flax seed into DHA for use by our brains.

Omega 3 fats
e.g. alpha-linolenic acid in flax seed, and EPA and DHA in fish

Anti-inflammatory compounds
e.g. prostaglandin E1, resolvins and protectins

Omega 3 and 6 are essential polyunsaturated fats that our bodies require from our diet. A problem occurs when we consume excessive quantities of omega 6 compared to omega

3 fats. This is because, as mentioned above, they compete with each other for use in our cells. Interestingly, arachidonic acid, produced from omega 6 oils, can sometimes be converted to anti-inflammatory compounds called lipoxins. This may occur with the consumption of aspirin and salicylic acid (natural aspirin) in plants. Omega 9 fats, such as the monounsaturated oleic acid in olive oil, avocados and macadamia nuts, are also thought to have anti-inflammatory properties.

Phytochemicals in fruit, vegetables, herbs and spices complement omega 3 and 9 fats in reducing inflammation, by inhibiting two compounds critical in the inflammatory process: NF-κB and the enzyme COX-2. Phytochemicals that inhibit the activation of NF-κB include capsaicin in capsicums and chillies, curcumin in turmeric, diallyl disulfide in garlic, kaempferol in apples and berries, piperine in pepper, polyphenols in ginger, quercetin in onions and tomatoes, resveratrol in red wine and grapes, and sulforaphane in broccoli and cabbages (Anand *et al.* 2008; Devi *et al.* 2015; Shishodia *et al.* 2005; Winters & Kelley 2017), see Figure 5.1.

Many phytochemicals inhibit the actions of the COX-2 enzyme (with several inhibiting both NF-kB and COX-2), including diallyl disulfide in garlic, diosgenin in fenugreek, eugenol in cloves, gingerols in ginger, kaempferol in apples and berries, and oleocanthal in olive oil (Anand *et al.* 2008; Beauchamp *et al.* 2005; Devi *et al.* 2015; Zhang *et al.* 2017).

Sirtuin 1 (also called sirt 1) is a protein within our cells that has many functions, including influencing the replacement of cells and glucose metabolism, and has been suggested to be involved in longevity. Sirtuin 1 also inhibits the inflammation-promoting action of NF-kB (Cori *et al.* 2016). Several phytochemicals are known to promote sirtuin 1, including resveratrol in grapes and red wine, and curcumin from turmeric.

Compounds similar to prostaglandins, called isoprostanes, are additional inflammatory molecules. They are formed without

COX enzymes, through the oxidation of fats, especially arachidonic acid from omega 6 fats. Polyphenols from cocoa and dark chocolate, and red wine, can reduce isoprostane production (Croft 2016).

We can gauge the role of phytochemicals in reducing inflammation by noting their effect on the levels of compounds in our blood and urine that indicate inflammation in our body. Consuming cherry extracts has been shown to reduce levels of several inflammation indicators (interleukin-6, C-reactive protein and uric acid) in blood samples taken following high intensity cycling and marathon running (Howatson *et al.* 2010; Bell *et al.* 2014). The researchers credited this to the anthocyanins in cherries. By limiting uric acid production, cherries can help lower the incidence or severity of the painful inflammation condition, gout.

Drugs that inhibit the inflammatory cytokine, tumour necrosis factor-alpha (TNF-alpha), are effective in treating osteoarthritis, rheumatoid arthritis and other inflammatory diseases (Aggarwal *et al.* 2013; Hess *et al.* 2011; Toussirot & Wendling 2007). Several phytochemicals are known to reduce levels of TNF-alpha. These include asiaticoside from the herb gotu kola, curcumin in turmeric and gingerol in ginger (He *et al.* 2011; Mashhadi *et al.* 2013; Jiang *et al.* 2017). One study involving over one hundred people found eating various herbs and spices for a week reduced levels of inflammation indicators, such as TNF-alpha, in samples of their blood (Perceval *et al.* 2012). Eating spices also limited DNA damage in their blood samples that were subsequently treated with the free radical-forming hydrogen peroxide. Groups of ten to 12 participants ate less than 3 grams daily of different herbs and spices for the week. Spices showing particular anti-inflammatory potency were cloves, cumin, ginger, paprika (i.e. dried chillies) and turmeric, as did the herb rosemary. Several small clinical trials have demonstrated the anti-inflammatory properties of

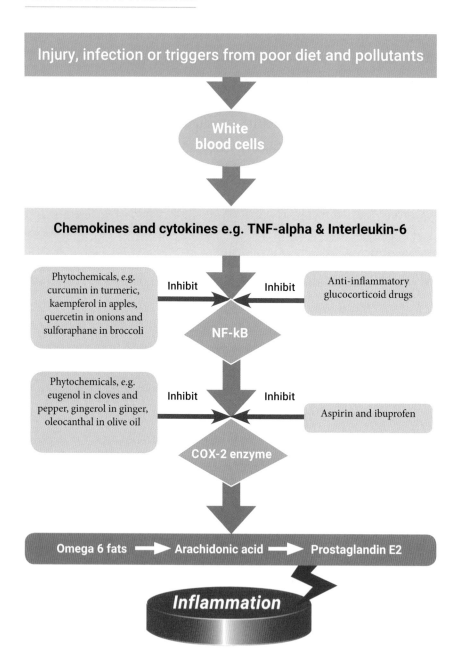

Figure 5.1. Diagrammatic representation of the NF-κb:COX-2 path to inflammation and the stages where drugs and phytochemicals inhibit its progression.

curcumin, from turmeric, lead to tangible relief from arthritic pain (e.g. Kuptniratsaikul *et al.* 2009; Chandran *et al.* 2012).

Uterine fibroids (uterine leiomyoma) are benign tumours, a common and sometimes painful condition for women and thought to be at least partly resulting from inflammation. A trial of 33 women with uterine fibroids found drinking a green tea extract (equivalent to about five cups of green tea per day) for four months, significantly reduced the size of the fibroids (Roshdy *et al.* 2013).

Aspirin is a drug commonly used for the management of inflammatory pain. It is probably the most widely used artificial variant of a phytochemical, being a modified version of the natural plant compound salicylic acid, which is a polyphenol. Specifically, the aspirin molecule has the addition of a simple arm of two carbon and five hydrogen atoms (an acetyl arm) attached to salicylic acid, which is thought to make it less irritating on the stomach. The acetyl arm separates when absorbed from the stomach and small intestine into the blood, so that most effects of aspirin are due to salicylic acid, which is found in low doses in many fruits, vegetables, herbs and spices (Duthie & Wood 2011). Incidentally, the same group of scientists who developed aspirin added two acetyl arms to morphine. The laboratory volunteers who tested the new drug were said to feel so heroic after taking diacetylmorphine that they named the infamous compound heroin (Jeffreys 2008).

Given that aspirin has been a popular drug since the 1890s, it is surprising that it was not until the late 1960s to early 1970s that scientists gradually solved the mystery of how aspirin worked to reduce pain and fever (Vane 1971; Jeffreys 2008). Aspirin inhibits the action of COX enzymes (Vane & Botting 2003). As mentioned previously and shown in Figure 5.1, the COX-2 enzyme catalyses the production of prostaglandin E2, which causes inflammation. It also stimulates thromboxane, which promotes blood vessel constriction and blood clotting (Fitzpatrick 2004). As a consequence of inhibiting the COX-2 enzyme, aspirin reduces inflammation and thins the blood. A range of phytochemicals, including naturally occurring salicylic acid, produce health benefits through the very same process (see Figure 5.1).

Salicylic acid is concentrated in some plants, such as the bark of willow trees and the herb meadowsweet, from which salicylic acid was originally synthesised, but is ubiquitous amongst plants because it is crucial to plant defences. Some vegetables and spices contain detectable levels of salicylic acid and it is estimated that the average salicylic acid intake from food per day in the UK is about 4 milligrams (Duthie & Wood 2011). Some plants, especially spices, have a tangible amount of salicylic acid, with mint containing 5 mg per 100 grams, cumin containing about 3 mg per 100 grams, turmeric 2 mg per 100 grams (note a typical aspirin tablet contains 300 mg). Immature fruit can have quite high levels of salicylic acid and other compounds aimed at deterring animals from eating the fruit until the seeds ripen. This can cause stomach problems, when eating fruit picked too green (Hungerford 2012).

In addition to the salicylic acid in plants, many phytochemicals reduce inflammation by inhibiting the same enzyme as aspirin. As mentioned above, oleocanthal in olive oil drives down inflammation by inhibiting COX-2 enzyme, which is the same process by which aspirin and another pain-relieving drug, ibuprofen, operate (Beauchamp et al. 2005). Aspirin and ibuprofen both belong to the group of drugs called non-steroidal anti-inflammatories. Phytochemicals in ginger, such as gingerol, also reduce inflammation by inhibiting the COX-2 enzyme. In a study examining the capacity of ginger to reduce inflammation after intense exercise, half of 74 participants who consumed two grams of ginger (either raw or heated) daily for eleven days reported less pain following exercise than those taking a placebo (Black *et al.* 2010). Associated with the diminished perception of pain, those taking ginger had lower levels of prostaglandin E2 in their blood, the inflammatory compound produced by COX-2. There is additional evidence that ginger phytochemicals (gingerols and shogaols) reduce inflammation by also inhibiting lipoxygenase (LOX) enzymes that produce leukotrienes, which is another pathway to inflammation (Grzanna *et al.* 2005). Aspirin does not provide this avenue to lowering inflammatory pain, whereas ginger supplies a multi-pronged attack on inflammation.

It is worth noting the potential inflammatory-related effects of several plant compounds called lectins, oxalates, phytates and saponins. These are made by plants as defence compounds, with lectins and phytates concentrated in seeds, and oxalates and saponins spread throughout plants, including in the leaves (Heldt & Piechulla 2011). Lectins, oxalates, phytates and saponins can potentially promote intestinal damage, with some lectins involved in leaky gut, allowing them to enter the blood stream. Lectins and phytates may promote inflammation in some people because our immune system can interprete them as foreign molecules and instigate an inflammatory response (de Punder & Pruimboom 2013). Lectins include gluten and wheat germ agglutinin. A range of different lectins are reasonably abundant in grains, legumes such as beans, peanuts and soybeans, and nightshade plants such as tomatoes and eggplants. Fruit picked while green can also contain a high concentration of lectins, because the compounds help to restrain animals from eating fruit until seeds are ripe. Phytates are particularly abundant in legumes such as beans and soybeans. Oxalates are common in kale, purslane, soybeans and spinach, while saponins are present in many plants in minor concentrations, but are relatively abundant in quinoa and soybeans.

Lectins, oxalates, phytates and saponins can bind to sugars and minerals and are sometimes referred to as antinutrients because they can reduce nutrient absorption from our gut. Oxalates, for example, bind to calcium and can accumulate in crystals that can cause painful arthritis-like symptoms. However, there is some evidence that low levels of lectins, oxalates, phytates and especially saponins, may be associated with health benefits in some people, such as providing anti-microbial effects, reducing cholesterol levels, removing excessive metals and potentially contributing to reducing cancer risk (He *et al.* 2018).

A good proportion of lectins and phytates can be removed by soaking seeds in water and/or sprouting or fermenting the seeds, and a fair amount decompose when cooked (Schlemmer *et al.* 2009; Heldt & Piechulla 2011). However, some people may find they are simply better off avoiding some plants that contain lectins or phytates such as wheat, legumes or tomatoes and other nightshade plants. Oxalates can be reduced a little by cooking, though saponins, which are probably the least problem, are less easily removed or degraded.

In summary, unresolved chronic inflammation is a very serious health issue. It damages healthy tissue and contributes to pain and many diseases including allergies, arthritis, heart disease, some cancers and dementia. A significant cause of inflammation is the protein NF-kB, which triggers the production of the COX-2 enzyme; this in turn catalyses inflammatory compounds from omega 6 fats.

Phytochemicals help switch off chronic inflammation by blocking the actions of NF-κB and inhibiting the enzyme COX-2. This mode of action is the same as produced by some pain-relieving drugs, such as aspirin and ibuprofen. Phytochemicals that inhibit inflammation include curcumin in turmeric, diallyldisulfide in garlic, eugenol in cloves, gingerol in ginger, kaempferol in apples, oleocanthal in olive oil and sulforaphane in broccoli and cabbages. Hesperetin in citrus and quercetin in apples, citrus, onions and tomatoes help relieve hay fever and other allergy symptoms by limiting the over production of histamine.

Chapter 6

Phytochemicals and fibre contribute to maintaining a healthy weight

> ## KEY POINTS
>
> - Eating fruit, vegetables, herbs and spices, and drinking tea, helps achieve and maintain a healthy weight in several ways.
> - Fibre and healthy plant fats can satisfy hunger, reducing overeating.
> - Fibre and many phytochemicals feed healthy gut microbes, which are beneficial to weight management.
> - Fibre and several phytochemicals, such as anthocyanins in blueberries, catechins in tea and ellagitannins in raspberries and strawberries, reduce the rate of glucose absorbed from our food into the blood. Lowering blood glucose levels reduces insulin spikes, limiting the amount of glucose converted into fat, while helping allow the burning of fat.
> - Plants that contribute to weight management include avocados, blueberries, cabbages, capsicums, green tea, nuts such as almonds and macadamias, olive oil and strawberries.

Being overweight can be unhealthy, and makes manual tasks more difficult. Once our weight increases towards and into obesity, the risk of various diseases escalates considerably, especially heart disease, stroke, type 2 diabetes, dementia and some cancers (González-Castejón & Rodriguez-Casado 2011). Fat tissue contains a mix of fat cells (called adipocytes), connective tissue and immune cells. Fat tissue secretes cytokines, messenger compounds promoting inflammation, into the blood stream. They can also increase insulin resistance (González-Castejón & Rodriguez-Casado 2011). As a result, obese people can carry persistent chronic inflammation, which may cause ongoing pain and increase the risk of developing some diseases (Zhang & An 2007; Leiherer *et al.* 2013).

Being obese is often associated with several health issues, grouped together under the term metabolic syndrome. However, not all people with metabolic syndrome are obese. Metabolic syndrome combines several of the following conditions: abdominal obesity, insulin resistance and high blood sugar, elevated triglycerides (fats) in the blood, high blood pressure and low levels of high-density lipoproteins (HDLs, 'good' cholesterol). These characteristics are linked to increased rates of heart disease, stroke and type 2 diabetes (Basu *et al.* 2010; González-Castejón & Rodriguez-Casado 2011; Amiot *et al.* 2016).

Eating a range of fruit and vegetables helps achieve weight loss and maintain a healthy weight. This is partly because many plants are high in nutrients but low in calories, and their high fibre content fills us up. Fibre is essential food for healthy gut microbes, which help with weight management through the production of healthy short chain fatty acids such as butyrate (Mercola 2017).

Processed food such as white bread has had much of the plant fibre removed, reducing its ability to make us feel full and limiting the fibre available for the support of beneficial gut microbes. Highly processed food is also often low in some vitamins, other phytochemicals and/or minerals (Hungerford 2012). A diet dominated by processed rather than whole food probably causes a degree of malnourishment. This is thought to cause an urge to overeat, fuelled by our bodies' search for missing nutrients. Consuming a diet that includes a wide variety of fruit, vegetables, herbs and spices can help meet our nutritional requirements and can therefore help reduce the urge to overeat.

Avocados and many nuts, such as almonds and macadamias, are high in fibre and good fats that can reduce hunger. Olive oil contains a particularly healthy combination of fats, especially the monounsaturated fat oleic acid. In addition to reducing inflammation (described previously), using olive oil as a salad dressing helps to satisfy our hunger so that we don't eat too much.

Phytochemicals such as capsaicin and capsiate from chillies can also reduce appetite, while increasing our metabolic rate to help burn fat (Yoshioka et al. 1999; Aggarwal & Yost 2011; Ludy et al. 2011). The caffeine in coffee and tea may contribute marginally to weight management in some people, by helping to burn stored fats. Sulforaphane, found in broccoli and cabbages, can promote the development of brown or intermediate beige fat tissue. These tissues have more mitochondria (the energy processing factories within cells) than normal white fat cells and therefore burn more energy (Nagata et al. 2017).

Catechins, a group of flavonoids found in tea and in smaller concentrations in coffee, have also been shown to increase energy expenditure in some people (Baspinar et al. 2017). A study involving 35 people with metabolic syndrome found that the participants who drank four cups of green tea a day over eight weeks had greater weight loss, by an average of 2.5 kg, compared to those drinking hot water (Basu et al. 2010). Those drinking green tea also showed a decrease in oxidative damage to LDL 'bad' cholesterol, which contributes to atherosclerosis, and a better ratio of HDL 'good' cholesterol to LDL compared to people in the study who drank hot water (Basu et al. 2010). A separate study found improved weight loss by combining the consumption of catechins in tea with exercise (Maki et al. 2009). It is speculated that drinking tea, especially green tea, helps manage weight by lowering appetite and reducing glucose absorption from the gut, while increasing energy expenditure and fat burning (Rains *et al.* 2011).

Adiponectin is a protein that promotes fat burning. It is typically found in lower than normal concentrations in people with metabolic syndrome, and especially type 2 diabetes patients (Lihn *et al.* 2005). Curcumin, from the spice turmeric, may promote the secretion of adiponectin (Leiherer *et al.* 2013).

Angiogenesis, the process of growing new blood vessels around cells (described in more detail in Chapter 9 in regards to cancer), is an important process in the expansion of fat tissue, because fat cells require access to a blood supply. Compounds that prevent excessive angiogenesis, such as lycopene, which provides the red colour of ruby-red grapefruit, tomatoes and watermelons, can help reduce this process.

Calories and kilojoules are units used to measure the amount of energy provided by food. The source of calories influences the way that fat accumulates in our bodies. A principal cause of fat accumulation, and therefore weight gain, is thought to be prolonged periods of elevated insulin in our blood (Fung 2016). Insulin is a hormone produced in the pancreas in response to the presence of glucose (a type of sugar) in our circulation. Eating protein also raises insulin levels, but to lesser degree. Insulin travels through our blood, where it triggers cells to absorb glucose, convert glucose into fat (in liver cells), regulate amino acid metabolism from protein, and delay fat burning (Rodin 1985). The rapid drop in blood glucose associated with high insulin levels can make us hungry. Interestingly, eating fat only increases insulin levels marginally, if at all, which may help explain why olive oil and nuts keep us feeling full for longer.

Some glucose is present in most foods, and at moderate levels is a fundamentally beneficial nutrient for life. Our bodies can make glucose from proteins and fats when required. Glucose occurs as a latticework of linked molecules in bread and makes up half of each crystal of table sugar (sucrose). The other half of table sugar crystals is fructose, which in excess contributes to fat accumulation, insulin resistance and damages the liver and pancreas (Gillespie 2015; Fung 2018).

Consuming table sugar and other refined carbohydrates, such as white bread and fruit juice lacking fibre, promotes more rapid glucose absorption into the blood, and associated increased insulin release, than eating the same amount of calories from most unprocessed plants. Carbohydrates that rapidly raise blood glucose, and therefore insulin levels, have a high glycaemic index (GI). Most whole, unprocessed plants have a low GI due to their fibre and phytochemicals, which slow and limit the absorption of glucose into the blood stream. Exceptions include potatoes. Glycaemic load (GL) considers the impact of a serving of a particular food. Low GI food, and a low GL meal, are more beneficial for blood glucose levels and weight management.

The glucose in our blood that is not used immediately for energy is stored, some as a chain of glucose called glycogen, with excess converted to fat. The burning of fat is delayed until insulin levels fall. Fat within cells and ongoing high glucose levels in the blood lead to insulin resistance, meaning that it takes increased levels of insulin to trigger cells to remove glucose from the blood. This ultimately leads to type 2 diabetes (Fung 2018).

Constant high glucose levels in our blood cause damage through the formation of compounds called advanced glycation end products (AGEs). These AGEs are formed when glucose in the blood sticks to and damages proteins and fats, changing their function and making them act like free radicals. When the fats that make up cell membranes are damaged by glucose, the tightly governed entry into our cells is compromised. In addition, because proteins are a hugely diverse group of compounds, many aspects of metabolism can be affected by damage from

AGEs. AGEs are also thought to contribute to the thickening of blood vessel walls, causing an increase in blood pressure, and can lead to blindness when capillaries in the eye are affected. In addition to problems with high blood glucose, extended periods of elevated insulin may also contribute to cardiovascular disease, especially through atherosclerosis (Madonna & De Caterina 2009; Rensing et al. 2011; Fung 2018).

One of the most significant contributions to weight management by phytochemicals is their ability to lower blood glucose levels and reduce the rate, and perhaps the amount, of glucose absorbed from our food, thereby restricting both blood glucose and insulin levels. Human trials show that eating just a small amount of cinnamon can reduce blood glucose levels, as well as reducing LDL 'bad' cholesterol (Khan et al. 2003; Anderson et al. 2016). Cinnamon may also reduce the development of AGEs. This appears to be due to phytochemicals in cinnamon, especially methylhydroxychalcone, improving the effectiveness of insulin (i.e. increasing insulin sensitivity) and/or mimicking the role of insulin in triggering glucose uptake into cells (Jarvill-Taylor et al. 2001; Anderson et al. 2016).

Phytochemicals in chillies and capsicums also reduce blood glucose levels. After four weeks of adding 30 grams of chillies to their meals daily, blood insulin levels of 36 trial participants fell significantly (Ahuja et al. 2006).

The digestive enzyme alpha-amylase is found in saliva and in the small intestines. It breaks down starches, such as in bread, into glucose units to be absorbed into the blood. Eating raspberries, strawberries and sweet potatoes, and drinking tea, slows the absorption of glucose from food into the blood by reducing the amount of alpha-amylase produced in saliva and the small intestines (McDougall et al. 2005; Törrönen et al. 2012). Blueberries and blackcurrant can reduce glucose absorption into the blood by inhibiting the release of another digestive enzyme called alpha-glucosidase, which is produced in the lining of the small intestine (McDougall *et al.* 2005). Researchers found evidence that phytochemicals called ellagitannins in raspberries and straw-berries, and catechins in tea, were responsible for their inhibitory effect on alpha-amylase, while anthocyanins in blueberries were responsible for the inhibition of alpha-glucosidase (McDougall *et al.* 2005). Australian native bush foods, Davidsonia plums and leaves of anise and lemon myrtles, have also been found to inhibit alpha-amylase activity in laboratory studies (Konczak *et al.* 2012).

Some weight loss drugs mimic the actions of phytochemicals to inhibit glucose absorption. For example, one type of weight loss drug reduces glucose absorption by inhibiting the enzyme alpha-glucosidase (Fung 2016), the identical mechanism provided by anthocyanins in blueberries. Some scientists feel that type 2 diabetic drugs that inhibit glucose absorption (e.g. by inhibiting alpha-amylase or alpha-glucosidase) are most beneficial because they reduce both blood glucose and insulin levels (Fung 2018).

The absorption of glucose into the blood is also slowed by the binding of some flavonoids to starch in the intestine, reducing the breakdown of starch into glucose units (Takahama & Hirota 2018). For example, tea polyphenols bind to rice starch, reducing its diges-tion into glucose units, and slowing glucose absorption into the blood. Other flavonoids, hesperetin and naringenin found in citrus, also bind to starch, reducing the rate of digestion.

In addition to reducing glucose absorption, several spices have been found to reduce the absorption of fat into the blood, by inhibiting the actions of enzymes that digest fat (McCrea *et al.* 2015). These include cinnamon, cloves and turmeric.

Several phytochemicals can help to improve the sensitivity of cells to insulin (i.e. reduce insulin resistance) by stimulating the action of a protein called glucose transporter isoform 4 (GLUT4). GLUT4 is located inside cells. It responds to insulin by moving to a cell's surface to transport glucose into the cell. By helping stimulate this action, phytochemicals help reduce insulin resistance, therefore lowering the amount of insulin required to remove glucose from the blood into cells. Phytochemicals that have been found in laboratory studies to stimulate the action of GLUT4 include the anthocyanin, cyanidin 3-O-glucoside, found in blackberries, blueberries, plums and pomegranates, and two other types of polyphenols: protocatechuic acid, found in grapefruit, olives and onions, and gallic acid, which is found in bananas, sage and strawberries. Gallic acid is also found in the Australian native fruits Cedar Bay and Herbert River cherries (Sayem *et al.* 2018).

In summary, eating fruit, vegetables, herbs and spices, and drinking tea, can contribute to achieving and maintaining a healthy weight in several ways. Their fibre and healthy fats (especially in avocados, nuts and olive oil) help fill us up which makes us less inclined to overeat. Many phytochemicals, and the minerals that plants contain, may also help reduce the urge to overeat. Fibre and some phytochemicals slow glucose absorption, reducing insulin spikes, and feed healthy gut microbes that can help with maintaining a healthy weight. Beneficial phytochemicals include anthocyanins in blueberries, ellagitannins in raspberries and strawberries and methylhydroxychalcone in cinnamon.

Chapter 7
Phytochemicals and fibre feed gut microbes

KEY POINTS

- The term gut microbes refers to microorganisms, mostly bacteria and fungi, that live in our stomach and especially our intestines. Beneficial gut microbes help maintain healthy stomach and intestinal linings and produce favourable compounds such as B vitamins and short-chain fatty acids.
- Beneficial gut microbes eat the fibre we consume in plants.
- Many phytochemicals, such as anthocyanins in blueberries, catechins in tea and quercetin in citrus and onions, also promote beneficial gut microbes. In turn, gut microbes modify some phytochemicals, increasing their absorption into the blood.
- Plants and plant products containing phytochemicals that feed healthy gut microbes include apples, blueberries, citrus, dark chocolate, garlic, grapes, onions and tea.

In recent years we have become more aware of the significance of healthy gut microbes. These bacteria and fungi are important for maintaining stomach and intestinal health, through their role in producing many essential compounds. There are hundreds, even thousands, of different types of gut bacteria, some more beneficial to our wellbeing than others. They compete with each other, and the food we eat influences the balance between them. For example, garlic contains oligosaccharides (small chains of sugars) that stimulate the growth of healthy gut microbes (Reid 2016).

Fibre, which can only be sourced from plants, is the fundamental dietary ingredient necessary for maintaining healthy gut microbes. It includes non-soluble fibre, the stringy, thicker parts of plants that helps food pass through our digestive system; and soluble fibre, which absorbs water, becoming gel-like (Mercola 2017). Most fruit, vegetables, nuts and grains contain both insoluble and soluble fibre. We cannot digest fibre by ourselves. It is the gut microbes, concentrated in our large intestine (bowel) that use fibre as food. Gut microbes also eat resistant starch, which is often considered a third type of fibre. Starch is a network of glucose which plants make for energy storage, analogous to our glycogen and fat deposits. Resistant starch is a crystalised form of starch that is less easily digested (i.e. is resistant to digestion). Small amounts occur in various plants. Resistant starch also develops in starchy plant foods such as potatoes and rice, when they are cooled in the fridge after cooking (Enders 2015). In return for our providing gut microbes with fibre, resistant starch and shelter, they produce various compounds that are important to us, including several B group vitamins and short-chain fatty acids, which are a type of fat with small tails (Enders 2015; Morowitz *et al*. 2011). The short-chain fatty acids are used as fuel by cells in our intestines, and are anti-inflammatory compounds.

Butyrate is one of these important short-chain fatty acids. We absorb butyrate from some fats and oils, such as butter and ghee. Gut bacteria are an important source of butyrate, which they make in our large intestine by fermenting fibre from plants we eat. Butyrate provides many benefits that may include contributing to good mental health and to reducing the risk of developing colon cancer (Clarke *et al.* 2008; Saldanha *et al.* 2014; Bourassa *et al.* 2016).

Many phytochemicals have a stimulating effect on healthy gut microbes. In return, many gut bacteria are essential for modifying phytochemicals so that they are more easily absorbed into our blood and cells. For example, flavonoids in our food are typically attached to a molecule of glucose or other sugar (called a glycoside). An example is the flavonoid quercetin, which is often joined to two glucose molecules in the plant material we eat (this version is called rutin). Gut microbes split the sugar molecules off to release quercetin. Further splitting of quercetin can occur by bacteria in the gut, which leads to smaller polyphenol compounds that are better absorbed in the bloodstream (Williamson & Clifford 2010; Braune *et al.* 2016; Tomás-Barberán *et al.* 2017). Similarly, gut microbes in the large intestine convert ellagic acid from strawberries into smaller units that are absorbed into the bloodstream (Cardona *et al.* 2013).

The composition of gut microbe species influences the number of polyphenols that are made available for absorption from our intestines. Polyphenols, such as catechins from tea and proanthocyanidins from red wine, promote beneficial gut microbes (Cardona *et al.* 2013). Blackcurrant, dark chocolate and extracts from grape seeds can also promote beneficial gut bacteria, such as *Bifidobacterium* spp. and *Lactobacillus* spp. (Cardona *et al.* 2013). For example, a study with 20 people found drinking a chocolate extract with high levels of chocolate flavanols increased the growth of these good gut bacteria (Tzounis *et al.* 2011). Consuming a drink made from wild blueberries rich in anthocyanins was also found to increase *Bifidobacterium* spp. after a six week human trial (Vendrame *et al.* 2011).

Sulfoquinovose is a type of sugar bound to sulphur and found in the leaves of plants. It is abundant in leafy vegetables, especially parsley and spinach, and is an important source of fuel for beneficial gut bacteria (Speciale *et al.* 2016). It has recently been suggested that sulfoquinovose in leafy vegetables is useful for promoting beneficial bacteria over unhealthy bacteria (Huang 2016).

In summary, the fibre in plants we eat is essential food for beneficial gut microbes. Some phytochemicals also feed beneficial gut microbes, including catechins from tea, and polyphenols in dark chocolate, quercetin in apples, citrus and onions and sulfoquinovose in many leafy vegetables.

Chapter 8

Phytochemicals enhance our detoxification system

KEY POINTS

- Our liver and kidneys play a central role in removing toxins from our bodies. Phase 1 and 2 enzymes convert toxins for removal.
- Many phytochemicals enhance the phase 1 and 2 enzyme systems, promoting detoxification.
- Particularly beneficial detox-enhancing phytochemicals include catechins in tea, curcumin in turmeric, limonene and naringenin in citrus and sulforaphane in broccoli and cabbages.

We absorb toxins from air and water pollutants, and exposure to pesticides and other chemicals, as well as from some of the food we eat. Our bodies are constantly removing these toxins through our breath, faeces, sweat and urine.

Our bodies have developed sophisticated ways for detoxification. Our liver and kidneys provide the backbone of the response to toxins. The liver contains enzyme systems, described broadly as phase 1 and phase 2, that modify toxins to ensure they are eliminated through the faeces, or through urine via the kidneys.

The phase 1 detox system is based on a group of enzymes called CYP 450. These are concentrated in the liver but also occur in our lungs and brain. CYP 450 enzymes modify toxins to make them more soluble in water because our blood is water-based.

There are a range of CYP 450 enzymes that act on different groups of toxins. CYP 450 1A1, for example, is involved in the detoxification of carcinogens (cancer-causing compounds). Paradoxically CYP 450 1A1 occasionally activates carcinogens, such as the heterocyclic amine PhIP produced in meat when cooked at high temperatures (Androutsopoulos *et al.* 2009). There is evidence that some phytochemicals can inhibit the carcinogen inducing activities of CYP 450 1A1. These include galangin in the ginger-like plant galangal, kaempferol in apples and tea, and tangeretin in citrus, especially orange and lemon peels (Androutsopoulos *et al.* 2009).

Phase 2 enzymes such as glutathione-s-transferase continue the detoxification process by further modifying toxins and carcinogens. This makes them more water soluble, allowing them to be easily excreted (Gupta *et al.* 2014).

Several phytochemicals are known to assist with our bodies' natural detoxification process. For example, sulforaphane from cabbages and broccoli activate the protein Nrf2, which in addition to building antioxidants, is involved in detoxification by promoting the production of phase 2 detoxifying enzymes such as glutathione (Surh 2011; Gupta *et al.* 2014). The phytochemical limonene, which provides the citrus smell of lemons and oranges, stimulates the detoxification process, in both phase 1 and phase 2. Naringenin, a flavonoid found in citrus, especially grapefruit, can keep our livers healthy to perform detoxification processes, by reducing oxidation and inhibiting the transcription protein NF-kB that promotes inflammation (Hernández-Aquino *et al.* 2017).

Two Chinese studies of people exposed to air pollution found sulforaphane from broccoli enhanced the detoxification process. An initial pilot study involving 50 people for seven days, followed by a larger study looking at 291 people over 12 weeks, found drinking broccoli shoot extracts increased detox-ification in participants' bodies, as measured by excretion of air pollutants such as benzene in urine (Kensler *et al.* 2011; Egner *et al.* 2014).

A recent study shows that the flavonoid quercetin, found in apples, onions and tomatoes, increases the lifespan of honey bees exposed to pesticides by 9-20%, suggesting an important role of quercetin in detoxifying pesticides (Liao *et al.* 2017).

In summary, phytochemicals that enhance the removal of toxins include curcumin in turmeric, galangin in galangal, gingerol in ginger, kaempferol, limonene, naringenin and tangeretin in citrus, plus sulforaphane in broccoli and cabbage.

Chapter 9

Phytochemicals contribute to reducing the risk of developing some cancers

---

KEY POINTS

- Phytochemicals can help inhibit the development, survival and spread of some cancers, such as breast, prostate and colon cancers. These phytochemicals include carotenoids, such as lycopene in tomatoes, polyphenols especially from berries, citrus, flax seed, tea and turmeric, and sulphur compounds in cruciferous vegetables (e.g. broccoli and cabbage), garlic and onions.
- The processes by which phytochemicals contribute anti-cancer benefits include:
  - promoting the excretion of carcinogenic compounds
  - inhibiting the growth of new blood vessels around tumours (therefore reducing tumour growth)
  - inhibiting inflammation-enhancing proteins that can promote cancer
  - enhancing the antioxidant capacity of cells to reduce free radical damage
  - promoting cancer cell death (apoptosis).

The World Health Organization estimates that between a third and half of cancer cases are preventable through good lifestyle choices, such as not smoking tobacco, limiting alcohol use, regularly exercising and eating plenty of fruit and vegetables. For example, a 2002 report estimated that not eating enough fruit and vegetables was responsible for around 19 per cent of gastrointestinal cancers (e.g. stomach and colon cancers; World Health Organization 2002). Around 38 per cent of deaths from cancer in Australia during 2013 were thought to be attributable to life style factors, such as smoking, and not eating sufficient fruit and non-starchy vegetables; suggesting around 16,700 deaths could be prevented annually in Australia through lifestyle changes (Wilson *et al.* 2018). That is a lot of people who could continue enjoying their lives.

Cancers are diverse and complex. The term cancer refers to abnormal cells that are growing and multiplying out of control, although some tumours get to a point and lie dormant. Oxidative stress from free radicals can cause damage to our mitochondria (the energy producing units found in each cell) and DNA, contributing to the initiation, development and spread of cancers (Li *et al.* 2016). Maintaining healthy mitochondria is critical to protecting against cancers, and damaged mitochondria are thought by some to be the key instigators of cancer development (Seyfried 2015; Christofferson 2017). Flavonoids can promote the removal of damaged mitochondria (Galati & O'Brien 2004).

Chronic inflammation is also linked to the establishment and progression of cancers. Several inflammatory cytokines (such as interleukin-6 and TNF-alpha) and the inflammation-initiating protein NF-κB are known to be involved in cancer development and spread (Li *et al.* 2016). NF-kB can reduce the effectiveness of cancer treatments by inhibiting cancer cell death (Yoon & Liu 2007). Blocking inflammatory cytokines and NF-κB can therefore reduce the growth of tumour cells, making them more sensitive to anti-cancer agents (Gupt *et al.* 2017). Phytochemicals in pomegranates and the flavonoid tangeretin in citrus peel have been shown to reduce NF-kB levels in breast cancer tissue in rat studies (Gul *et al.* 2017). Limonene, the oil in orange and lemon peels that provides the smell of citrus, has also shown some cancer inhibiting properties in laboratory tests (Miller *et al.* 2011). Research has demonstrated that limonene is absorbed into fat tissue after a month of consuming citrus juice that includes the peel, or taking limonene concentrate for two to six weeks (Miller *et al.* 2010; 2013). The latter trial demonstrated that limonene had accummulated in breast tissue, with the potential to contribute to limiting cancer development.

Surprisingly, many of us carry around minute dormant tumours, less than a millimetre in size. Autopsies of people who died from accidents or other reasons unrelated to cancer, indicate about a third of middle aged women have microscopic tumours in their breast and a similar proportion of men have microscopic tumours in their prostate (Folkman & Kalluri 2004). These minute tumours can't grow unless they have access to a direct blood supply from new blood vessels around the tumour, providing oxygen and nutrients (Folkman & Kalluri 2004). The growth of new blood vessels is called angiogenesis.

Tumour cells trigger angiogenesis by promoting proteins called vascular endothelial growth factor (VEGF) and/or plate-let-derived growth factor (PDGF). The stimulation of new blood vessels by VEGF and PDGF provides an essential role in wound healing and general growth, but has negative consequences when the process is hijacked by tumours. Various metabolic pathways are inter-related, with the inflammation-promoting enzyme COX-2 able to cause the production of VEGF (Gately & Li 2004). As described earlier, many phytochemicals inhibit COX-2, such as gingerol in ginger and oleocanthal in olives.

Therefore, a central aspect of being able to prevent and treat cancer is the management and inhibition of unrestrained angiogenesis. Many phytochemicals possess anti-angiogenesis properties. Ellagic acid, found in several fruit especially berries, has been shown to reduce angiogenesis around tumours in a laboratory experiment, by inhibiting the production of VEGF and PDGF to the same degree as at least one cancer drug (Labrecque *et al.* 2005). Ellagic acid can also help detoxify or remove carcinogens by enhancing phase 2 detoxification enzyme activities (Sakulnarmrat 2012). Cinnamon has been found to reduce VEGF in mice, probably due to the phytochemicals procyanidins and cinnamaldehyde (Zhang *et al.* 2017). The lycopene in tomatoes is anti-angiogenic, with the potential to inhibit the development of new blood vessels around tumours (Wilkinson 2015). Broccoli, and other plants in the cabbage family, ginger and turmeric can also help inhibit angiogenesis (Kim *et al.* 2014; Wilkinson 2015).

Motivated by the knowledge that cigarette smoke contains carcinogenic compounds, Japanese researchers made a surprising discovery in the 1970s. They found potentially carcinogenic compounds in the smoke and charred surface of cooked meat (Nagao *et al.* 1977; Sugimura *et al.* 1977 - cited in Sugimura 1997). Cooking meat at high temperatures, such as by grilling and frying, causes the production of compounds called heterocyclic amines. These nitrogen-containing compounds are potential human carcinogens, and their abundance is correlated with colon, breast, prostate and pancreatic cancers (Monti *et al.* 2001; Weisburger 2002). Marinating meat with herbs and spices such as rosemary and turmeric, can reduce the production of heterocyclic amines during cooking, probably due to the antioxidant properties of their various phytochemicals (Monti *et al.* 2001; Aggarwal & Yost 2011; Salazar *et al.* 2014). Polyphenols, such as those found in tea, may also diminish the damage caused by heterocyclic amines, by reducing cell multiplication and/or promoting cancer cell death (Weisburger 2002).

The process of apoptosis (programmed cell death) in tumour cells is also central to cancer treatment. Polyphenols, such as resveratrol in grapes and red wine, and epigallocatechin-3-gallate in green tea, can promote apoptosis in tumour cells (Galati & O'Brien 2004; Grabacka *et al.* 2014). Ginger and turmeric, including curcumin extracts, and the sulphur compound PEITC in plants of the cabbage family, also promote cancer cell apoptosis (Gupta *et al.* 2014b; Kim *et al.* 2014; Wilkinson 2015).

Turmeric seems to help prevent cancer development, at least in part, by the ability of its key phytochemical, curcumin, to block the gene transcription factor NF-kB. This reduces the production of inflammatory compounds such as prostaglandin E2 (Wilkinson 2015). Recent laboratory research has found curcumin also selectively inhibits a protein in our cells called DYRK2 (Banerjee *et al.* 2018). DYRK2 activates another protein called proteasome 26s which is involved in removing damaged proteins from cells. By blocking DYRK2, and therefore inhibiting proteasome 26s, curcumin causes the accumulation of damaged proteins which can lead to the death of a cancer cell (Béliveau 2018). Some cancer drugs work by inhibiting proteasomes, and this research indicates curcumin has the potential to provide anticancer benefits through the same action.

Avocados contain an unusual type of fat called avocatin B, which has been found in a laboratory study to selectively target and destroy acute myeloid leukemia cells (Lee *et al.* 2015). Tomatoes may reduce the oxidation of prostate tissue, therefore perhaps help in the treatment of prostate cancer (Flores-Perez & Rodriguez-Concepcion 2012).

Several human studies have found that regular consumption of garlic, leeks and onions is associated with lower rates of cancers, especially of the oesophagus, stomach and colon. Consuming garlic extracts for a year was found to reduce the number and size of recurring colon adenomas (polyp pre-cursers to colon cancer) in a trial involving 37 patients (Tanaka *et al.* 2006). Eating broccoli at least once a month was associated with improved survival rates in bladder cancer patients (Tang *et al.* 2010). These benefits appear to be due to the blocking of tumour growth by their sulphur phytochemicals, allicin and diallyl sulphide in garlic and onions, and sulforaphane in broccoli (Fleischauer & Arab 2001; Béliveau & Gingras 2014). Garlic extract may also improve the immune system of cancer patients by increasing the activity of natural killer immune cells (Ishikawa *et al.* 2006), which are special white blood cells involved in eliminating viruses and tumours.

A protein within our cells called p53 is involved with suppressing cell cycles and promoting apoptosis. Defective p53 fail to cause the death of abnormal cells, which can lead to cancer. Curcumin from turmeric, ellagic acid in berries, epigallocatechin-3-gallate in green tea and tangeretin in citrus peels have all been found to activate p53, promoting the death of cancer cells in laboratory trials (He *et al.* 2011; Dong *et al.* 2014; Riaz *et al.* 2017).

A UK research team headed by Professors Gerry Potter and Dan Burke has made an exciting discovery regarding the anti-can-cer properties of some phytochemicals. They found an enzyme that seems to be largely restricted to cancer cells. Laboratory trials indicate the enzyme, CYP1B1, appears to transform some phytochemicals (which Potter, Burke and their team call salves-trols) into compounds that promote the death of cancer cells. The enzyme CYP1B1 is not present in healthy tissue (or is only at negligible levels), therefore salvestrol phytochemicals are only converted into lethal compounds in cancerous cells (Schaeffer 2012). Further research is required to confirm the consistency of these results and understand the process, but small case studies suggest encouraging outcomes in cancer treatment, especially due to the natural sources of these phytochemicals and their selectivity towards cancerous cells (Schaeffer *et al.* 2010).

Salvestrol phytochemicals found to interact with CYP1B1 are manufactured within plants to defend themselves against insects and pathogens. They include some polyphenols found in avocados, basil, blueberries, broccoli, grapes, mangoes, mulberries, olives, parsley and strawberries (Schaeffer 2012). For example, resveratrol from grape skins is used by CYP1B1 to make the compound piceatannol, which is toxic to cancer cells (Potter & Burke 2006). Because salvestrols are plant-defence phytochemicals, plants that need to protect themselves from insects and fungi while growing (e.g. organic produce, which is not protected by synthetic pesticides) are thought to have higher densities of salvestrols (Schaeffer 2012).

In their book, *Foods to Fight Cancer*, Béliveau & Gingras (2017) point to studies showing regular consumption of soybeans, and fermented products such as miso and tofu, is linked to lower incidents of breast and prostate cancers. However, they note that purified and concentrated isoflavone supplements do not necessarily provide these benefits, and may sometimes increase cancer risk. Genistein, the isoflavone in soybeans as well as chickpea, has been seen in laboratory studies to have a similar action to the anticancer drug tamoxifen. Both appear to block the growth of tumours by reducing the amount of oestrogen attaching to and apparently promoting growth in pre-cancerous cells, especially in breast tissue (Béliveau & Gingras 2017).

Skin cancers, melanoma and non-melanoma (including basal cell and squamous cell carcinomas), killed around 2,000 Australians in 2015, according to the Cancer Council of Australia (https://www.cancer.org.au/about-cancer/types-of-cancer/skin-cancer.html). Recent research indicates that, in addition to the general anti-cancer benefits of eating and drinking fruit, vegetables, herbs and spices, applying some phytochemicals to the skin may provide some protection against UV-induced non-melanomas (Montes de Oca *et al.* 2017). In particular, the antioxidant and anti-angiogenesis properties of epigallocatechin-3-gallate in green tea may help reduce skin tumour expansion when applied to the skin. Feeding pomegranate extract to mice has also been found to reduce skin tumours (Montes de Oca *et al.* 2017).

The studies and processes described here offer good evidence that phytochemicals are beneficial in helping prevent the development of several cancers. Australians in general are not taking full advantage of these preventative benefits of fruits, vegetables, herbs and spices. However, we must be cautious when considering the degree to which phytochemicals can treat existing cancer. Once cancer has developed, medical intervention is essential. Further studies are still required to determine the role of phytochemicals, such as curcumin in turmeric, in cancer management (Gibson-Moore & Spiro 2017). Phytochemicals are likely to be more effective at helping inhibit cancer development, than killing off large existing tumours. They may, however, play an important role in enhancing the success of medical treatments and reducing the chance of recurrence. For example, the sulphur phytochemical PEITC in plants of the cabbage family has been found to improve the activity of some cancer drugs (Gupta *et al.* 2014).

In summary, phytochemicals can inhibit the growth of new blood vessels around tumours, therefore helping reduce cancerous tumour growth. These compounds include ellagic acid found in several fruits, especially berries, lycopene in tomatoes, sulforaphane in broccoli and other plants in the cabbage family, gingerol in ginger and curcumin in turmeric.

Phytochemicals can also promote the death of cancer cells. These include curcumin in turmeric, epigallocatechin-3-gallate in green tea, gingerol in ginger, resveratrol in grape skins and red wine and sulphur phytochemicals in garlic, onions and plants of the cabbage family. Some research suggests an enzyme called CYP1B1 is concentrated in cancer cells and is largely absent from healthy cells. This enzyme appears to transform some phytochemicals (which a British research team call salvestrols) into toxic compounds that promote the death of cancer cells in laboratory trials. Phytochemicals can support cancer therapies and recovery. Sulphur compounds in cabbage family plants can improve the benefit and activity of some cancer drugs.

Chapter 10

Phytochemicals contribute to cardiovascular health

KEY POINTS

- Phytochemicals help maintain the health of our cardiovascular system, reducing the chance of experiencing heart disease and stroke, and improving blood flow, which also benefits brain function. Key phytochemicals include beta-sitosterol in avocados, sulphur compounds in garlic, onions and the cabbage family, resveratrol in grapes and red wine, and polyphenols in apples, citrus, dark chocolate, ginger, olive oil, pomegranate, tea and turmeric.

- Phytochemicals contribute to cardiovascular health by:
  - increasing blood vessel flexibility and lowering blood pressure by promoting nitric oxide
  - inhibiting excessive aggregation of blood platelets to thin the blood
  - reducing oxidation damage to LDL 'bad' cholesterol and blood vessels
  - reducing inflammation of blood vessels

It is estimated that in 2014-15, 4.2 million Australian adults were suffering from some form of cardiovascular disease, including high blood pressure, coronary heart disease or recovering from a stroke (AIHW 2017). According to the Heart Foundation of Australia, over 45,000 Australians died of cardiovascular disease in 2015, with nearly half a million hospitalisations in 2014 and 2015. That is far too many people! This high rate of cardio-vascular disease is shared by many other countries including New Zealand, the UK and US.

Cardiovascular health refers to the condition of the heart and blood vessels, with the latter influencing strokes. The World Health Organization estimates that inadequate consumption of fruit and vegetables was responsible for around 31 per cent of ischaemic heart disease (caused by reduced blood supply through atherosclerosis) and 11 per cent of strokes worldwide (World Health Organization 2002).

Eating a Mediterranean diet with abundant olive oil, fruit, nuts, vegetables and fish, is repeatedly associated with lower rates of cardiovascular disease (Grosso *et al.* 2017). For example, a Spanish trial of the Mediterranean diet followed 7,447 people at risk of cardiovascular disease for almost five years. They found consuming a Mediterranean diet with supplementation of either additional extra virgin olive oil (to around 50 ml per day), or extra nuts (30 grams daily), led to fewer incidents of heart attacks and strokes compared to participants who lowered their fat intake and consumed more bread, pasta, potatoes and rice (Estruch *et al.* 2013).

A recent study of nearly 2,000 Italians found that the more flavonoids they consumed from fruit and vegetables, the lower their risk of heart disease (Ponzo *et al.* 2015). A Japanese study following 40,000 adults over 11 years found people who regularly drank green tea had a lower incidence of cardiovascular disease (Kuriyama *et al.* 2006). A Finnish study examining the diets of 3,932 adults found that those who ate the most fruit and vegeta-bles, especially citrus and cruciferous vegetables (e.g. broccoli) had the lowest incidence of stroke (Mizrahi *et al.* 2009). A review of eight studies, involving a total of 257,551 people, concluded that eating five servings of fruit and vegetables daily would likely provide a significant decline in the number of strokes worldwide (He *et al.* 2006).

Certain lifestyle changes have been demonstrated to significantly improve indicators of cardiovascular health. For example, a trial involving 35 patients with coronary atherosclerosis (narrowing of blood vessels supplying the heart) found that the 20 participants who undertook lifestyle changes had dramatically improved cardiovascular health (Ornish *et al.* 1998). The lifestyle changes involved eating a vegetarian diet low in fat (10% of total calories), participating in stress management training (e.g. meditation) and group support meetings, and engaging in moderate aerobic exercise. The one patient who was a smoker quit smoking at the start of the trial. The 20 patients following the lifestyle changes had reduced artery clogging (measured as percentage stenosis) from an average of 41.3% of the artery diameter at the start of the trial, to 38.5% after just one year and down to 37.3% after five years (Ornish *et al.* 1998). In comparison, participants not undertaking the lifestyle changes had an increase in artery clogging (from 40.7 to 51.9% after five years), plus more angina pain and cardiac events.

In a similar study, 23 non-smoking cardiac patients who undertook the lifestyle improvements detailed above had increased blood flow after only three months, whereas comparative patients not undertaking lifestyle changes had a decrease in blood flow (Dod *et al.* 2010).

Plants play a key role in studies showing improved cardiovascular health in people eating Mediterranean diets, or undertaking lifestyle changes. Phytochemicals from plants, especially those in apples, citrus, garlic, grapes, leafy vegetables, olive oil, pomegranate, spices and tea, contribute to improved cardiovascular health in several ways. They provide strong antioxidant and anti-inflammatory effects, promote blood vessel flexibility and blood flow which reduces blood pressure, lower blood platelet aggregation (i.e. they reduce clots and thin the blood), maintain healthy cholesterol and homocysteine levels, enhance healthy gut microbes and help in weight management. Improving and maintaining cardiovascular health has flow-on benefits for a healthy brain and retaining men's erectile function.

Elevated levels of the amino acid homocysteine are associated with cardiovascular disease. This is thought to occur, at least in part, by homocysteine inhibiting nitric oxide formation in the body and therefore reducing blood vessel dilation by nitric oxide (La & Kan 2015). It may also lead to blood platelet clumping and atherosclerosis. A 16 week trial with cardiovascular disease patients found that half of participants (38 people) reduced their homocysteine levels, as well as lowering their blood glucose and insulin, by consuming a daily meal with whole grains (brown rice and barley), legume powder and small amounts of onions and pumpkin (Jang *et al*. 2001). The researchers noted the benefits were associated with increases in beta-carotene, lycopene and vitamin E levels in the patients' blood. The other 38 participants in the trial who ate refined rice instead of whole grains etc., showed no significant changes in homocysteine, glucose or insulin levels. Another study assessing data from 938 healthy adults confirmed the benefits of whole grains in reducing homocysteine levels (Jensen *et al*. 2006).

Phytochemicals help reduce the amount of fat and glucose that we absorb from our food, and balance cholesterol levels. For example, a small study of six people found that including 14 grams of mixed spices (cinnamon, garlic, ginger, pepper and turmeric) and the herb rosemary with a high fat meal, reduced the absorption of fat into the blood stream (McCrea *et al*. 2015). This was associated with evidence that the spices inhibited the actions of fat digesting enzymes; cinnamon, cloves and turmeric being the most potent enzyme inhibitors. A further study found consuming 1 to 6 grams of cinnamon daily for 40 days reduced blood triglyceride levels by 23-30% and LDL 'bad' cholesterol levels by 7-27% (Khan *et al.* 2003).

The phytochemical beta-sitosterol, found abundantly in avocado flesh and present in olive oil and macadamia nuts, reduces the absorption of cholesterol from our diet and lowers the production of cholesterol by our liver (Duester 2001). It is important to note that many researchers consider it is not simply the total amount of LDLs (i.e. low density lipoproteins which transport fats and cholesterol through our blood) or total cholesterol contained within LDLs, that are critical factors in cardiovascular health. The amount of LDLs that are damaged by oxidation appears to be a primary issue (Libby 2006). Having a high ratio of HDLs, which return fats and cholesterol to the liver, relative to LDLs also seems important for good cardiovascular health. Drinking green tea and consuming olive oil have been found to encourage a healthy ratio of 'good' HDL cholesterol to LDL 'bad' cholesterol (Basu *et al.* 2010; Covas 2007).

Human trials have shown that phytochemicals from a range of plants can reduce the oxidation damage to LDL 'bad' cholesterol. For example, eating strawberries can decrease oxidative damage to LDLs and thin the blood (Alvarez-Suarez *et al.* 2014; Basu *et al.* 2009). Polyphenols in olive oil and pomegranate juice also protect LDLs from oxidation (Covas 2007; Aviram *et al.* 2004). A European study with 200 participants found that those who consumed 25 mL of olive oil containing high polyphenol levels daily for three weeks reduced their oxidative damage to LDLs (Covas *et al.* 2006). Consuming 20 mL of olive oil each day for six weeks has also been found to reduce protein biomarkers that are indicators of cardiovascular disease (Silva *et al.* 2015).

There is accumulating evidence that the combination of oxidation and inflammation is central to the development of cardiovascular disease. If we do not have enough antioxidants circulating in our blood, oxidative damage to fats and cholesterol in LDLs can trigger inflammation. This damages blood vessel walls and can lead to atherosclerosis (Li & Fang 2004; Libby 2006). An excessive consumption of omega 6 processed seed oils, such as from corn, soybeans and sunflower seeds, combined with a low omega 3 fat intake, such as from fish and flax seed, has been implicated in cardiovascular disease (Ramsden *et al.* 2010). This is thought to be due to oxidation of LDLs (especially from eating lots of deep fried food), increased blood clotting and inflammation (Kummerow 2014; Hyman 2016; Sun *et al.* 2019).

C-reactive protein is a critical indicator of inflammation and raised levels in the blood are associated with cardiovascular disease. Researchers have found that reducing the levels of this protein can lower the number of heart attacks (Li & Fang 2004; Libby 2006). Consuming cherries and strawberries has been found to reduce C-reactive protein levels in people's blood (Bell *et al.* 2014; Edirisinghe *et al.* 2011). Eating apples, plants in the cabbage family, onions and turmeric provide phyto-chemicals that can inhibit the transcription protein NF-kB that instigates inflammation (refer to Chapter 5 for more details on inflammation).

New research suggests inhibiting the protein NF-kB has benefits to cardiovascular health beyond lowering inflamma-tion. A study using mice as subjects has found that inhibiting NF-kB reduces calcium-related thickening and stiffening of arteries (Peterson *et al.* 2018).

Phytochemicals can help reduce the build-up of blood vessel plaques and reduce vessel wall thickening. In one small but remarkable trial, drinking pomegranate juice reopened narrowed carotid arteries by around a third. Ten people with severe carotid artery stenosis (narrowing of the carotid arteries in the neck by 70-90%, typically due to atherosclerosis) drank 50 mL of pomegranate juice daily for one year. At the end of the year, the narrowing of their neck arteries had reduced by an average of 35%, that is the channels within their arteries had widened (Aviram *et al.* 2004). They also showed reduced blood pressure. Another nine patients who drank a placebo rather than pomegranate juice developed a further 9% increase in carotid artery blockage by the end of the year (Aviram *et al.* 2004). The authors suggested that the benefits of pomegranate juice were likely due to the antioxidant properties of the pomegranate polyphenols, including anthocyanins.

A larger study involving 289 people found drinking 240 mL of pomegranate juice daily for up to 18 months slowed the progression of carotid artery thickening. This finding applied, however, only to participants with the most severe signs of cardiovascular disease, and not those with less severe symptoms (Davidson *et al.* 2009). Another trial found improved blood flow, with less symptoms of ischaemia (reduced blood flow to the heart) during exercise or other stress tests, in heart disease patients who drank pomegranate juice for three months. In contrast, ischaemia progressed over the three months in the other half of the 45 trial patients who did not drink pomegranate juice (Sumner *et al.* 2005).

There is evidence that garlic can slow atherosclerosis and perhaps sometimes reverse plaque buildup. For example, 27 adults with metabolic syndrome who took aged garlic extracts daily for an average of 345 days showed reductions in blood vessel plaque (Matsumoto *et al.* 2016).

Around a third of US adults over the age of 40, surveyed in 2011-12, reported taking aspirin or a similar blood thinning medication, as a cardiovascular disease preventative (Gu *et al.* 2015). There is still debate around the pros and cons of regular, preventive use of aspirin. It is thought to help people of high cardiovascular disease risk, especially those who have previously had a heart attack, but does potentially increase the risk of excessive bleeding, including hemorrhagic stroke (Halvorsen *et al.* 2014; McNeil *et al.* 2018). Aspirin thins the blood by inhibiting the action of COX enzymes (Vane & Botting 2003). The COX-2 enzyme, which promotes inflammation, also catalyses the production of thromboxane, which promotes blood vessel constriction and blood clotting (Fitzpatrick 2004). Many phytochemicals thin the blood by the same mechanism as aspirin, that is, by inhibiting the COX-2 enzyme. This includes the flavonoids hesperetin found in citrus and quercetin in apples, onions and tomatoes (Guo *et al.* 2014). These phytochemicals are not absorbed at the same concentration as many drugs, so that they may not provide the same degree of blood thinning as aspirin. However, regular consumption of plants containing these phytochemicals can be of practical value and typically provide no side effects, often delivering multiple benefits.

The omega 3 fat EPA, abundant in fish and produced in our bodies after we eat the plant-sourced omega 3 fat ALA, also thins the blood (Dyerberg *et al.* 1978). As an example, five men consuming 40 grams of flax seed oil daily for 23 days showed reduced blood clotting (Allman *et al.* 1995). This appeared to be due to the omega 3 ALA in flax seed converting to EPA within blood platelets, which thinned the blood. A further six men in the trial who consumed 40 grams of sunflower seed oil, containing the omega 6 linoleic acid, did not show any improved blood clot response. The omega 3 fat ALA may also help reduce atherosclerosis. An American study evaluating 1,575 participants found the higher the level of ALA consumed, the less plaque thickness was seen in their carotid arteries (Djoussé *et al.* 2003).

A review of twenty human trials concluded that garlic typically lowers systolic blood pressure (the first or upper number indicating the pressure of blood when the heart contracts) by an average of 5.1 mm Hg and diastolic blood pressure of 2.5

mm Hg (Reid 2016). A greater reduction in blood pressure (8.7 mm Hg systolic; 6.1 mm Hg diastolic) from garlic was evident in people with high blood pressure. The mechanism appears to be the sulphur phytochemicals in garlic releasing hydrogen sulfide, which can stimulate blood vessel relaxation. There is also evidence, from animal studies, that piperine from pepper can lower blood pressure by limiting calcium entry into blood vessel walls, thereby relaxing blood vessels (Taqvi *et al.* 2008).

Some phytochemicals, such as catechins in tea, also improve blood flow. For example, blood vessel dilation was observed within two hours of drinking either black or green tea, in a study involving twenty-one women. Associated with this, long term tea drinking (both black and green teas) reduces blood pressure (Liu *et al.* 2014). A trial of 19 adults with high blood pressure found that drinking black tea twice daily for eight days significantly reduced their blood pressure (Grassi *et al.* 2015). It appears that the tea polyphenols (especially catechins and theaflavins) stimulate nitric oxide to relax the blood vessel muscles (Jochmann *et al.* 2008).

A small but steady production of nitric oxide helps keep blood vessels flexible and therefore maintains normal blood pressure, although rapid production of high levels of nitric oxide in blood vessels during septic shock can cause danger-ously low blood pressure (Villanueva & Giulivi 2010). Human trials have found that eating spinach or drinking beetroot juice, which are good sources of nitrates that can be converted to nitric oxide, reduce blood pressure by a modest but potentially important amount (Gee & Ahluwalia 2016).

A study involving 45 healthy adults demonstrated increased blood flow and reduced blood pressure after eating dark choco-late or drinking sugar free cocoa, as a result of increased nitric oxide production in blood vessels (Faridi *et al.* 2008). This can have practical applications, one example being for scuba diving. In a study of 42 divers, half of the participants who ate 30 grams of dark chocolate 90 minutes before a dive showed improved blood vessel dilation. This was associated with increased levels of nitric oxide in their blood, reducing the stress of diving on their circulatory system (Theunissen *et al*. 2015).

There have been multiple human trials demonstrating the value of the DASH diet (Dietary Approaches to Stop Hypertension) in lowering high blood pressure. The DASH diet promotes the consumption of abundant fruit (around four serves a day), vegetables (four serves a day), nuts (one to two serves a day) and whole grains, poultry and fish with reduced saturated fats, low fat dairy and low salt (Sacks *et al*. 1995; Sacks & Campos 2010). One of the many DASH diet trials involved 459 people, some with high blood pressure. Results showed that those who ate just fruit and vegetables lowered their bood pressure more than those who ate a standard western diet, and the people who ate a DASH diet had the greatest lowering of their blood pressure (Appel *et al*. 1997). Another trial with 412 participants found that the DASH diet reduced blood pressure compared to a standard western diet, especially where sodium (table salt) was reduced (Sacks *et al*. 2001). The naturally occurring nitrates and nitrites in fruit and vegetables, which convert to nitric oxide to relax blood vessels, are thought to be a significant aspect of the DASH diet's ability to lower blood pressure (Hord *et al*. 2009; Bryan *et al*. 2010).

There is also evidence that quercetin, a flavonoid found in many fruit and vegetables, including apples, oranges and onions, can reduce blood pressure. A trial involving 93 overweight adults found that consuming concentrated quercetin in capsules (150 mg) daily for six weeks significantly lowered systolic blood pressure (by an average of 2·6mm Hg) and reduced oxidative damage to LDL 'bad' cholesterol (Egert *et al*. 2009). The amount of daily quercetin intake (150 mg) in that trial can be sourced by eating 100 grams each (i.e. 400 grams in total) of kale, red onion, watercress and wild rocket

(Bhagwat & Haytowitz 2015). Another study involved 19 adults with prehypertension and 21 participants with stage 1 hypertension, taking a higher amount of quercetin in capsules (730 mg) daily for 28 days. Interestingly, blood pressure fell in participants with stage 1 hypertension, but not in those with prehypertension (Edwards *et al.* 2007).

In summary, cardiovascular disease cuts short the lives of too many Australians and people around the world. However, eating abundant fruit, vegetables, herbs and spices, and drinking tea, can reduce the chance of developing cardiovascular disease. Phytochemicals contribute to improved cardiovascular health by providing strong antioxidant and anti-inflammatory effects. They promote blood vessel flexibility to reduce blood pressure and increase blood flow, reduce blood platelet aggregation to thin the blood, maintain healthy cholesterol and homocysteine levels, enhance healthy gut microbes and help in weight management.

Human trials have found phytochemicals from olive oil, pomegranate juice and strawberries can reduce oxidation damage to LDL 'bad' cholesterol. There is some evidence that consuming garlic and pomegranates may help slow atherosclerosis and perhaps reverse plaque build-up. Many phytochemicals thin the blood by the same mechanism as aspirin, that is by inhibiting the COX-2 enzyme. This includes the flavonoids hesperetin found in citrus and quercetin in apples, onions and tomatoes. Eating beetroot, dark chocolate and garlic, and drinking tea lowers blood pressure by increasing nitric oxide levels, which relaxes blood vessel muscles. Quercetin can also reduce blood pressure.

Chapter 11

Phytochemicals boost brain and nerve function, helping to prevent dementia and relieve anxiety and depression

---

KEY POINTS

- Eating abundant fruit and vegetables is associated with better mental performance, lower levels of anxiety and depression, and reduced risk of developing dementia.

- Phytochemicals in fruit, vegetables, herbs and spices improve our mental wellbeing through their antioxidant and anti-inflammatory benefits, as well as maintaining blood flow to the brain.

- Anthocyanins in berries, carnosol in rosemary and sage, curcumin in turmeric, lutein in spinach, oleocanthal in olive oil, other polyphenols in citrus and dark chocolate, resveratrol in grapes and sulforaphane in cabbage family vegetables are particularly beneficial.

Consuming a diet that includes plenty of vegetables can help lower your chance of developing dementia and declining brain function, according to a US study on the development of dementia in 3,718 people aged 65 years and older (Morris *et al.* 2006). Other studies support this trend, including a recent evaluation of the diets of nearly one thousand people in the Northern Manhattan Study, where eating abundant fruit and vegetables, plus lower intakes of red meat and associated 'western diet' foods, were linked to better cognitive performance (Gardener *et al.* 2017). Data from the long-term Nurses' Health Study suggests that older people who eat blueberries and strawberries display a slower decline in cognitive performance (Devore *et al.* 2012).

Maintaining blood vessel health and blood flow to the brain by eating plants is critical for mental performance. A recent study found people with high blood pressure showed early signs of damage to brain tissue and reduced cognitive performance (Carnevale *et al.* 2018). Indeed, vascular dementia results from strokes, ministrokes or tiny blockages in blood vessels around the brain.

Oxidative stress and inflammation are significant contributing factors in the development of degenerative brain diseases such as dementia (Corbi *et al.* 2016). The inflammation process described earlier (see Chapter 5), driven by chemical messengers called cytokines which activate the protein NF-kB, damages brain cells. Many phytochemicals decrease inflammation within the brain by inhibiting the activation of NF-kB (Corbi *et al.* 2016). These include anthocyanins in blueberries, curcumin in turmeric, kaempferol in apples, quercetin in onions, resveratrol in grape skins and sulforaphane in broccoli and cabbages. Activation of sirtuin 1 by phytochemicals, such as resveratrol and sulforaphane, can also lower inflammation and reduce the death of nerve cells induced by beta-amyloid peptide (Corbi *et al.* 2016). On the other hand, diminished sirtuin 1 activity is linked to lower protection of nerve cells.

Flavonoids including anthocyanins in blueberries, as well as curcumin from turmeric, can improve neuron signalling within our brains and may help increase nerve cell size within the hippo-campus (Flores 2017). The hippocampus is a region of the brain involved in memory, learning and emotions. Phytochemicals can promote or maintain levels of a protein called brain derived neurotrophic factor (BDNF), which enhances the growth and survival of brain neurons, and has an important role in learning and memory by promoting connections between brain cells (Whyte *et al.* 2016). There appears to be an association between low BDNF levels and abundant beta-amyloid peptide, the compound that clogs the brains of Alzheimer's disease sufferers. Research suggests oleocanthal from olive oil and curcumin from turmeric can inhibit the formation of beta-amyloid plaques in the brain, and perhaps even help clear them (Abuznait *et al.* 2013; Tang & Taghibiglou 2017).

Maintaining good cardiovascular health is important for reducing the risk of developing vascular dementia and Alzheimer's disease. As mentioned earlier, vascular dementia results from poor blood flow into sections of the brain. There is also an association between maintaining good blood flow to capillaries throughout the brain and the build up of beta-amyloid plaques. Blood flow provides oxygen and nutrients to brain cells and removes wastes. It is not yet clear whether beta-amyloid plaques develop because too much beta-amyloid peptide is produced or whether poor blood supply cannot remove sufficient waste peptide from around brain cells - possibly both (Furman 2018).

An abundance of insulin, the hormone that triggers the extraction of glucose from the blood into cells, can also limit the degradation of beta-amyloid peptide. After insulin has prompted the removal of glucose from the blood, it is degraded by insulin-degradation enzyme. This enzyme is also involved in degrading beta-amyloid peptide, so that the more insulin that is required to be degraded, the less insulin-degradation enzyme is available for removing excessive beta-amyloid peptide (Farris *et al.* 2003; Bredesen 2017). Therefore, too much sugar in the diet can trigger too much insulin, which probably hinders the removal of excess beta-amyloid peptide. This then increases the risk of developing and progressing Alzheimer's disease (Bredesen 2017). If glucose is present at high levels in the blood for long periods, it can also damage blood vessels, reducing blood supply across the brain.

People suffering an infection can often experience a gloomy mood; this is called sickness behaviour. There is evidence that sickness behaviour is caused by inflammatory cytokine messengers spreading from the infection to the brain to influence mood (Chang *et al.* 2009; Bullmore 2018). Indicators of inflammation, such as C-reactive protein, have been found to be elevated in some people suffering from anxiety and depression (Wium-Andersen *et al.* 2013).

Anxiety and depression are serious mental health disorders that appear to be increasingly common. Several large studies have found a diet with abundant fruit, vegetables and fish are linked to lower incidents of anxiety and depression (Jacka 2019). Phytochemicals can contribute to easing depression and anxiety. A study over 10 years looking at the dietary intakes of 82,643 women in the Nurses' Health Study, found that there were fewer incidents of depression in women eating the highest levels of flavonoids (Chang *et al.* 2016). An Australian trial found improving the diet can help lower depression symptoms in just twelve weeks (Jacka *et al.* 2017).

One recent study found that people with generalised anxiety disorder (GAD, characterised by uncontrollable excessive worrying) had a higher ratio of pro-inflammatory to anti-inflammatory cytokines in their blood compared to people who did not have anxiety. Specifically, those suffering anxiety had elevated levels of the inflammation-promoting cytokines TNF-alpha and interferon-y (IFN-y) compared to the inflammation-resolving cytokines interleukin-4 (IL-4) and IL-10 (Hou *et al.* 2016). Stress and social pressures clearly have a role in some episodes of depression and anxiety. Interestingly, there is evidence that stress, such as public speaking, can increase the levels of pro-inflammatory cytokines (e.g. IL-6) and therefore inflammation (Bellingrath *et al.* 2013; Bullmore 2018).

Some antidepressant drugs, such as Prozac, appear to work by inhibiting the breakdown or reabsorption of the neurotransmitter serotonin, therefore helping keep its levels elevated. This suggests that low levels of serotonin can play a role in anxiety and depression. The amino acid tryptophan is a building block for serotonin production. Inflammatory cytokines promote the conversion of tryptophan into a compound called kynurenine, instead of serotonin, so that elevated levels of inflammatory cytokines can reduce serotonin levels. Inflammation in the brain can also damage brain cells, including neurons (Bullmore 2018).

Drugs that reduce inflammation have been found to provide anti-depression benefits. In one example, a study summarised the results of seven human trials involving 2,370 patients. Those who were given drugs to reduce pro-inflammatory cytokines experienced reduced feelings of depression compared to patients who took placebos (Kappelmann *et al.* 2016). Phytochemicals such as curcumin in turmeric, gingerol in ginger and sulforaphane in broccoli, which help reduce inflammation, may therefore help reduce anxiety and depression symptoms in some people.

A trial involving 22 young men and teenagers (average age of 17) with autism spectrum disorder plus a history of behavioural problems found improvements after participants took daily sulforaphane capsules produced from broccoli sprouts (Singh *et al.* 2014). The participants taking sulforaphane showed reduced irritability and improved social interactions, in contrast to people who took a placebo not containing sulforaphane. The researchers suggested that the benefits may be due to sulforaphane's capacity to stimulate the body's antioxidant glutathione (via Nrf2 promotion) and contribute to the removal of toxins.

A recent study involving 21 people aged 18 to 21, and 50 children aged 7 to 10, found drinking blueberry extracts increased positive feelings and mood (Khalid *et al.* 2017). The herb sage improves memory and mood by slowing the degradation of the attention-promoting neurotransmitter acetylcholine (Tildesley *et al.* 2005; Kennedy *et al.* 2006).

Flavonoids in dark chocolate also appear to improve both memory and mood (Rendeiro *et al.* 2015). In addition to flavonoids, chocolate contains the amino acids phenylethylamine and tyrosine, which can improve mood by promoting the neurotransmitter dopamine. Some antidepressant drugs contain modified versions of phenylethylamine. Chocolate also stimulates the release of the neurotransmitter serotonin (Aggarwal & Yost 2011). The oft-heard comment about needing chocolate to cope with life's crises may contain more than a hint of truth!

Consuming omega 3 fats from flax seed, purslane and fish contribute to a healthy brain by reducing inflammation. The omega 3 fat DHA is a component of brain and nerve cell membranes. We consume DHA by eating fish and to a lesser degree, grass-fed animals, and a small proportion of the plant-sourced omega 3 fat ALA is converted into DHA. Good levels of DHA provide flexibility to neurons and improve transmission between brain cells (Morris 2018). Deficiencies in DHA are linked to anxiety and dementia. A recent study using rats as subjects found curcumin from turmeric increased the conversion of the flax-sourced ALA into the brain-active DHA (Wu *et al.* 2015).

Following a traumatic head injury, brain cells can be injured through oxidative damage from free radicals and inflammation (Prasad 2015). The oxidative damage to brain tissue impacts on the levels of BDNF (brain derived neurotrophic factor), reducing its ability to maintain healthy brain cells and their connections that allow learning and memory. Feeding rats curcumin from turmeric after mild traumatic injury reduced oxidative damage to brain cells and promoted BDNF levels, resulting in improved mental performance (Wu *et al.* 2006). Feeding rats omega 3 fats from fish oil also maintained BDNF levels (Wu *et al.* 2004).

Some phytochemicals, for example curcumin and sulforaphane, provide direct antioxidant benefits to brain cells. The activation of the protein Nrf2 by many phytochemicals also stimulates the production of powerful antioxidants within our cells (glutathione and SOD), contributing significantly to reduced oxidation in the brain.

Evidence from studies on mice suggests that the phytochemical carnosol, found in rosemary and sage, can reduce oxidative damage to mitochondria in brain cells following brain trauma, by promoting Nrf2 activity (Miller *et al.* 2015). The catechins in green tea have been found to reduce the oxidation damage to fats in the hippocampus, and to lower free radical levels in the hippocampus and cortex regions of the brain (Haque *et al.* 2008). Other phytochemicals such as resveratrol may contribute to the recovery of brain tissue after stroke or brain injury (Lopez *et al.* 2015). Flavonoids, such as catechins in tea and quercetin in apples and tomatoes, help increase blood flow, and this aids in healing.

Several phytochemicals can rapidly improve alertness and mental performance in people of any age. Coffee contains the alkaloid caffeine (as do chocolate and tea, in lower concentrations) which is one of the world's favourite stimulants. Caffeine improves mental alertness through its effect on several neurotransmitters in the brain. We feel more alert because caffeine can block access to brain cell receptors by adenosine. Adenosine makes us feel drowsy, and by blocking adenosine's access to brain cells, caffeine keeps us alert (Brunning 2015). Caffeine complements this by increasing the availability or responsiveness of dopamine receptors, allowing more of the neurotransmitter dopamine to communicate feelings of plea-sure and reward (Volkow *et al.* 2015).

Other phytochemicals boost our brains' performance. Researchers in a New Zealand study found improvements in the cognition of 36 adults who drank blackcurrant juice. They linked the improvement with reduced activity of a blood platelet compound called monoamine oxidase-B (MAO-B) and increased concentration of a compound called dihydroxy-phenylglycine (Watson *et al.* 2015). Overactivity of MAO-B is found in late onset Alzheimer's disease patients, while increased dihydroxyphenylglycine concentration is associated with improved memory.

A UK study involving 21 children aged 7 to 10 found improved word recall and recognition within several hours of drinking a wild blueberry drink (equivalent to eating 120 grams of wild blueberries). Even better results were seen after drinking juice containing the equivalent of 240 grams of blueberries (Whyte *et al.* 2016). Drinking wild blueberry juice for 12 weeks was also found to improve word recall tests and reduce depression symptoms in nine people with early signs of memory decline (Krikorian *et al.* 2010). Another UK study found improved mental alertness in 22 men who drank orange juice with added orange pomace, the by-product of juicing which contains fibre and flavonoids, especially hesperidin (Alharbi *et al.* 2016).

Carotenoids also have a positive effect on brain function. In particular, the amount of lutein and zeaxanthin present in the blood is correlated to better cognitive function (Renzi-Hammond *et al.* 2017; Khan *et al.* 2018). That is, people who regularly eat plants and/or eggs containing lutein and zeaxanthin tend to have better brain performance. A trial involving 51 young adults found supplementing the diet with 10 mg of lutein and 2 mg of zeaxan-thin daily for a year improved spatial memory (Renzi-Hammond *et al.* 2017). This amount of lutein and zeathanthin is present in a little over half a cup of cooked spinach. Consuming lutein and zeaxanthin have also been shown to improve the speed at which adults process visual information (Bovier & Hammond 2015).

Consuming abundant fruit and vegetables is associated with a lower chance of suffering from Parkinson's disease. The flavonoid tangeretin in citrus fruit (concentrated in the peel) may be beneficial in reducing nerve damage associated with Parkinson's disease (Vauzour *et al.* 2010).

In summary, anthocyanins in blueberries, oleocanthal from olive oil, other polyphenols in citrus, strawberries and turmeric, and sulforaphane in cabbage family plants, can help slow the development of dementia. Consuming broccoli, blueberries, dark chocolate and sage provide phytochemicals that can help reduce anxiety and depression and perhaps contribute to improved mental performance.

Chapter 12
Phytochemicals protect our eyes

KEY POINTS

- Eating fruit and vegetables containing the carotenoids beta-carotene, lutein and zeaxanthin provides essential antioxidant protection to our eyes. This reduces the chances of developing cataracts and macular degeneration.
- Plants containing good amounts of these carotenoids include corn and dark green leafy vegetables such as kale and spinach, plus broccoli, capsicum, citrus and tomatoes.

Our eyes come under daily bombardment from the high energy of light. The oxidative damage to our eyes is a significant contributor to cataracts and macular degeneration. It is analogous to the continuous light-induced oxidative attack on chloroplasts in plant leaves. Chloroplasts are compartments within plant cells where photosynthesis occurs. They contain chlorophyll molecules which provide their green colour. Due to their exposure to energy from sunlight, chloroplasts are highly susceptible to oxidative damage. Plants protect them from damage by interspersing antioxidant phytochemicals (especially beta-carotene and lutein) amongst chlorophyll molecules, within the chloroplast. Other antioxidants, especially glutathione, provide additional support. The cells in our eyes are protected in a remarkably similar way.

The cells within our eyes, including the lens, actively incorporate the antioxidant carotenoids lutein and zeaxanthin. Beta-carotene, which our bodies use to make vitamin A, also contributes antioxidant benefits to our eyes. These carotenoids are common in carrots, corn, dark green leafy vegetables such as kale and spinach, as well as broccoli, capsicum, citrus and tomatoes.

Studies have found that the more lutein and zeaxanthin in our diet, the lower the chance of developing cataracts and macular degeneration (Moeller *et al.* 2008). An Australian study looking at the eye health of 2,322 people over the age of 40, spanning a period of five years, found eating food rich in lutein significantly reduced the risk of developing nuclear cataract (the clouding of the centre of the eye lens; Vu *et al.* 2006). No clear effects of lutein were found on cataract development on the periphery and back of the lens, which the researchers thought may have been because there were fewer of these cases in their study.

A trial involving 108 people suffering early stages of macular degeneration examined supplemention with 20 mg of lutein, or 10 mg each of lutein and zeaxanthin, taken daily for 48 weeks. The results showed improved macular pigment and indicators of vision (Ma *et al.* 2012). A meta-analysis summarising eight trials involving 1,176 patients with macular degeneration confirmed the benefits of lutein and zeaxanthin for improving clarity of vision (Liu *et al.* 2015). Consuming 20 mg combined total of lutein and zeaxanthin daily is realistic, being equivalent of about 200 grams of cooked spinach, kale or mustard greens (USDA 2018).

Lutein and zeaxanthin protect our eyes through their antioxidant properties, and because they filter blue light (Ma *et al.* 2010). Interestingly, our exposure to blue light is not just from sunlight. Computers, mobile phones and LED lights all bombard our eyes with blue light. Perhaps there is an even greater need for lutein and zeaxanthin in the electronic age.

Our eyes use the antioxidant glutathione to boost the protection from carotenoids. Phytochemicals, such as sulforaphane from broccoli and cabbages, induce the gene transcribing protein Nrf2 to promote the production of glutathione within eye lens cells, which can reduce oxidative damage that leads to cataracts (Batliwala *et al.* 2017).

In summary, the carotenoids beta-carotene, lutein and zeaxanthin protect our eyes through their antioxidant properties, and because they filter blue light. Phytochemicals such as sulforaphane from broccoli and cabbages stimulate the production of the antioxidant glutathione to boost antioxidant protection of our eyes.

Chapter 13
Details of phytochemical groups

It would have been frustratingly impossible for early plant scientists to determine the chemical structures and precise roles of many phytochemicals. They were finally able to make progress once usable radio-isotope techniques were developed in the 1950s. The details of key plant physiological processes, such as photosynthesis, were not clarified until the carbon 14 isotope was available. While normal carbon atoms have a molecular weight of 12 (from 6 protons and 6 neutrons), carbon 14 atoms have 6 protons and 8 neutrons. Andrew Benson and Melvin Calvin's team used carbon 14 to follow the fate of carbon molecules through the photosynthesis process. This allowed the opportunity to follow 'labelled' atoms in carbon dioxide, through a series of chemical reactions, into a sugar molecule produced as the end result of photosynthesis.

While progress was being made in deciphering the chemical secrets of plants in the 1950s to 70s, scientists thought that most phytochemicals were of little use and simply waste products from plant metabolism (Hartmann 2007). Modern scientific equipment and techniques such as high performance liquid chromatography, mass spectrometry and nuclear magnetic resonance have allowed greater efficiency in determining active compounds and biochemical pathways. These techniques have shown the significant role played by phytochemicals in plants and people.

The link between high fruit and vegetable intake and lower rates of heart disease and cancer was becoming apparent in the 1960s. This focused research onto determining the compounds in plants that provide health benefits. It coincided with an understanding of the role of free radicals in disease.

One of the first focal points was the correlation between reduced cancer rates with consumption of beta-carotene, the orange pigment in carrots, and its ability to act as an antioxidant (Hercberg 2005). Sadly, taking concentrated supplements of purified beta-carotene has sometimes been linked to an increased risk of cancer (Hercberg 2005). This highlights the benefits supplied by the full mix of phytochemicals at concentrations found in whole plants, compared to purified, concentrated supplements of a single phytochemical. Daily consumption of fruit, vegetables, herbs and spices brings a constant supply of beneficial phytochemicals, steadily providing their health benefits, provided via a cascade of cell responses. We don't notice most of the cell responses triggered by plant chemicals, but tangible examples are the cool sensation we perceive from eating mint, and the heat from chillies, both of which are due to phytochemicals stimulating receptors on our cell membranes. As we have seen in Chapter 2, phytochemicals can be classified into six broad groups (see Figure 13.1), with most vitamins also considered as additional phytochemicals:

Alkaloids contain nitrogen but have a different structure to the amino acids that make up proteins. Examples of alkaloids are caffeine in coffee and tea, capsaicin found in chillies and theobromine in chocolate. These alkaloids act as stimulants and appear to increase the metabolic rate of some people, potentially helping to burn fat. The alkaloid capsaicin may reduce the perception of pain.

Alkaloids function as the front line, high powered chemical defence of many plants. Several of the alkaloids that we enjoy in low concentrations, such as caffeine in coffee and theobromine in chocolate, have a role as insecticides in plants. Alkaloids are present in the white milky sap of various plants such as rubber trees. Many alkaloids are highly toxic to people, such as the poison strychnine from the appropriately named *Strychnos nux-vomica*. Other alkaloids, such as morphine and quinine, provide us with high value medicines.

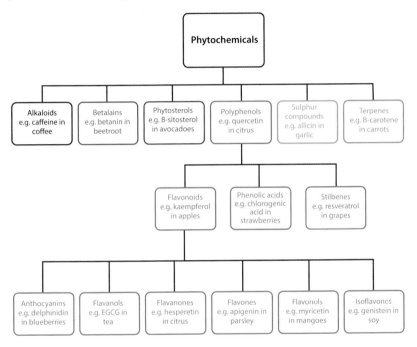

Figure 13.1 Broad groups of phytochemicals that provide health benefits. Note that the polyphenols have a diverse range of health-promoting phytochemicals; subgroups are shown.

B e t a l a i n s provide a yellow to red colouration to flowers and other plant parts including the red of beetroots, from which they derive their name. They are also found in prickly pear cactus and dragon fruits. Like alkaloids, betalains contain nitrogen, though have a different chemical structure. Examples are betanin and indicaxanthin. Betalains have a direct antoxidant capacity and also promote our cells to produce the strong anti-oxidant, glutathione. They can help protect LDL 'bad' cholesterol from oxidative damage and inhibit inflammation (Butera *et al.*

2002; Esatbeyoglu *et al.* 2015). Consuming betalain rich beet-root juice can lower the pain of osteoarthritis (Pietrzkowski *et al.* 2010). Betalains may even contribute to lowering blood pressure by increasing nitric oxide (Esatbeyoglu *et al.* 2015).

Phytosterols are chemically related to cholesterol and are found in seeds of various plants, especially legumes, nuts and whole grains such as sorghum. They include coumestrol in peas, soybeans and spinach and matairesinol in flax seed, broccoli and strawberries, as well as beta-sitosterol and campesterol in avocados, macadamia nuts and onions. Some phytosterols can interact with cell receptors for the hormone oestrogen (Visioli *et al.* 2000). Studies with mice suggest they may contribute to lowering the risk of developing cancer, by helping promote cell death in tumours. For example beta-sitosterol is associated with lower oesophageal cancer rates (Shahzad *et al.* 2017). As phytosterols are similar in structure to cholesterol, they are thought to lower cholesterol levels by competing with cholesterol absorption from the gut (Ostlund 2002). The flavonoid subgroup, isoflavones such as genistein (found in legumes such as lentils and soybeans), have phytosterol properties.

Polyphenols are based on the compound phenol, which contains six carbon atoms joined into a ring structure. Polyphenols are abundant water soluble compounds within plants. They are degraded by fungi and bacteria in the soil but are more slowly decomposed than other organic matter, providing interest in their ability to maintain high soil organic concentrations (Min *et al.* 2015).

Polyphenols include the broad groups flavonoids, phenolic acids and stilbenes. Curcumin in turmeric, gingerol in ginger and lignans, such as pinoresinol in olive oil, are polyphenols that don't fit neatly into these groups. The term tannin usually refers to large complex polyphenols containing many units joined together, such as ellagitannins in pomegranate and proanthocy-anidins in berries.

Phenolic acids include chlorogenic acid found in apricots and broccoli, ferulic acid in dark chocolate and mulberries, gallic acid in blackberries and pomegranates, and p-coumaric in apples and olives. Many phenolic acids, such as caffeic acid in blueberries and coffee, have only a single phenol, rather than multiple or *poly-phenols*. Other phenolic acids, such as ellagic acid in grapes, peaches and strawberries, contain multiple phenols. These compounds may help delay the development of cancer by enhancing the body's ability to remove carcinogens and reduce the conversion of nitrogen compounds into carcinogenic nitrosamines (Napier 1998). Ellagic acid has been demonstrated to reduce the growth of new blood capillaries around tumours (Labrecque *et al*. 2005). Salicylic acid, the active compound in aspirin and found in many plants, is a phenolic acid which can reduce inflammation and thin the blood.

Stilbenes (stilbenoids) include resveratrol, pterostilbene and puniculagins. Resveratrol is the most commonly discussed stilbene, considered the main healthy component of red wine. Resveratrol is also found in small amounts in avocados, blueberries, dark chocolate, plums and of course grapes (Sayeed *et al*. 2017). Pterostilbene is found in almonds, blueberries and mulberries. Both resveratrol and the closely related pterostilbene can reduce inflammation, enhance cardiovascular health and can induce the death of cancer cells (Sayeed *et al*. 2017; Li *et al*. 2018).

Flavonoids are a large group of polyphenols that have a multiple carbon ring structure (C6-C3-C6). Most flavonoids in plant foods are joined to either acid-alcohol or sugars, and these compounds are called glycosides (Amiot *et al*. 2016). Common flavonoids consumed include apigenin in celery and parsley, delphinidin from blueberries and wine, catechins in tea, hesperetin in oranges and mandarins, kaempferol in apples and tea, myricetin in mangoes, coffee and tea, naringenin in grapefruit and oranges and quercetin in apples, grapes, broccoli, onions and tea (Somerset & Johannot 2008). The types of flavonoids differ in chemical structure and effect, providing subgroups.

Anthocyanins are a type of flavonoid that provide deep blue and purple colours, especially in the skins of fruit such as eggplant, blueberries and raspberries. They include delphinidin in blueberries. There is good evidence that anthocyanins provide antioxidant and anti-inflammatory effects that can help reduce the risk of developing cardiovascular disease, cancer and dementia (Chen *et al.* 2006).

Flavanols include a range of catechins, most commonly found in tea. This includes epigallocatechin-3-gallate (EGCG), which is concentrated in green tea. They provide significant human health benefits, including promoting the death of tumour cells. Catechins are readily absorbed into the blood and are detectable within three hours of drinking tea. They have been found within prostate tissue after patients consumed six cups of green tea daily for six weeks, and within skin tissue after three months (Wang *et al.* 2010; Clarke *et al.* 2016).

Flavanones include hesperetin and naringenin in citrus, the latter being especially abundant in grapefruit. Hesperidin is a glycoside form of hesperetin with a sugar molecule attached. These compounds can reduce the severity of allergic responses by lowering histamine release, and they enhance the benefits of vitamin C.

Flavonols are a particularly abundant subgroup of flavonoids. They include kaempferol, myricetin and quercetin. Kaempferol is found in apples, cumin, grapefruit, mangoes, raspberries, riberry (i.e. the Australian native fruit of *Syzygium luehmannii*), black tea, tomatoes and wine. Kaempferol inhibits the enzyme COX-2, which promotes inflammation. Kaempferol can also help relax blood vessels and is an antioxidant, reducing the oxidation of LDL 'bad' cholesterol (Devi *et al.* 2015).

Plants containing myricetin include capsicums, carrots, eggplant, ginger, lettuce, mangoes, parsley and potatoes. Myricetin can help reduce blood pressure, contribute to weight loss and help prevent atherosclerosis by limiting oxidation of 'bad' cholesterol (Salvamani *et al.* 2014). There is evidence, from studies using mice, that myricetin promotes the function of mitochondria (which produce energy) in muscle cells, improving physical endurance (Jung *et al.* 2017).

Quercetin is an important flavonol found in a large range of fruit and vegetables including apples, broccoli, citrus, lettuce, onions, strawberries and tomatoes (Sayeed *et al.* 2017). Quercetin is a strong antioxidant and can reduce inflammation including arthritis. It does this by inhibiting enzymes (i.e. COX-2 and lipo-oxygenase, LOX) that promote inflammatory compounds (Lakhanpal & Rai 2007). Quercetin can inhibit excessive production of histamine, which causes allergic reactions (Bischoff 2008). In this way, quercetin can help relieve the symptoms of hay fever, eczema, sinusitis and asthma (Lakhanpal & Rai 2007). It can also contribute to the relief of gout symptoms by inhibiting the production of uric acid, and thins the blood by inhibiting thromboxane (Lakhanpal & Rai 2007; Gui *et al.* 2014). Isoquercetin, which is a glycoside of quercetin, has been found to inhibit influenza A and B viruses in rodent trials (Kim *et al.* 2010). Quercetin benefits cardiovascular health by reducing atherosclerosis and inflammatory cardiovascular risk factors (human-CRP, SAA, fibrinogen; Kleemann *et al.* 2011).

Flavones include apigenin in celery and parsley, and luteolin in apples and strawberries. They can reduce the oxidation damage to LDLs and can stimulate our cells to produce the strong antioxidant glutathione.

Isoflavones are another type of flavonoid with similarities to the phytosterols. They include daidzein and genistein, which are found in legumes such as lentils, peas and soybeans. They can help manage cholesterol levels and possibly reduce symptoms of menopause in some women. There is also interest in their potential to reduce the risk of developing breast and prostate cancers.

Sulphur compounds include allicin in garlic, indol-3-carbonol (I3C) in kale and sulforaphane from broccoli and cabbage. Plants make sulphur compounds as toxins to inhibit herbivorous insects, but they provide health benefits to us at the concentrations found in a typical diet. These sulphur compounds are interesting in that most of them are stored within plants in an inactive state, as part of a larger parent compound, requiring transformation before they become active. When plant tissue is broken, an enzyme stored in a separate compartment within the cell mixes with the parent compound, producing the active sulphur phytochemical. This happens after an insect chews leaves or a chef chops up a pile of ingredients.

For example, the pungent smell of cut garlic results from the conversion of the parent compound alliin, via the enzyme alliinase, to the active phytochemical allicin. When onions are sliced, enzymes convert an amino acid sulfoxide into the tear-jerking sulphur compound propanethial s-oxide (Brunning 2015).

In broccoli, cell damage from cutting or chewing causes an enzyme called myrosinase to mix with the parent compound glucosinolate, splitting off the active phytochemical sulforaphane. Excessive heating damages the enzyme myrosinase, reducing the amount of active sulforaphane produced. It is therefore best to only steam broccoli and Brussels sprouts for a few minutes, rather than boiling them for longer. Sulforaphane can be detected in the blood two hours after ingestion, and any remaining in the blood that has not been absorbed into tissues is excreted within 24 hours.

Heat also damages the enzyme alliinase in garlic and onions. Therefore let sliced garlic and onions sit for several minutes before cooking, to allow the chemical conversion to occur.

Terpenes are a broad group of fat and oil soluble phytochemicals. They include carotenoids, xanthophylls, monoterpenes and triterpenes. Carotenoids include alpha- and beta-carotene (from which our bodies can make vitamin A), astaxanthin (the orange colouring of salmon, which originates from the algae they eat), beta-cryptoxanthin, lutein, lycopene (the red colouring of tomatoes) and zeaxanthin. Carotenes play an important role in plants, especially as antioxidants within cells involved with photosynthesis. They also provide numerous health benefits, including as key antioxidants in eye health and potentially in reducing the development of some cancers, such as prostate cancer.

Limonene provides the citrus smell of oranges and lemons and is concentrated in their peels. It is a type of terpene called a monoterpene and stimulates the detoxification process. Saponins are another type of terpene abundant in legumes and quinoa.

Carnosic acid, and the related carnosol (which is what carnosic acid becomes after it has given away a hydrogen atom), are unusual terpenes with a phenolic group, which means they can also be considered a polyphenol. They are found in rosemary and sage. Their antioxidant capacity is so high that they are used as a food preservative (Birtić *et al.* 2015). They are probably useful in reducing oxidative damage in high light and/ or dry conditions within rosemary, sage and related plants of the Mediterranean region (Birtić *et al.* 2015).

Some phytochemicals come to us through animal products, such as the orange carotenoids in egg yolks. Manuka honey has excellent wound healing properties, probably due to a compound called methylglyoxal, which develops in honey from the transformation of dihydroxyacetone in the nectar of flowers of tea trees, called manuka in New Zealand (*Leptospermum scoparium*).

VITAMINS

Plants are an excellent source of most vitamins, and numerous health benefits of plants are directly attributable to their vitamin content. Many vitamins can be considered a special group of phytochemicals, although some can also be provided to us by animals. Vitamin B12 is available in animal products, such as meat, eggs and milk, and some algae. Vitamin D, synthesised from a cholesterol-like compound when our skin is exposed to sunlight, has some minor food sources, mainly from animals. Vitamin K2 is mainly obtained from meat, dairy and eggs, plus fermented plants such as natto (fermented soy) and sauerkraut (fermented cabbage).

Vitamins are compounds that are essential to our health. They must be sourced from our food because our bodies cannot manufacture them (except for vitamin D). Many vitamins fulfil roles as so called 'co-enzymes'. These compounds ensure that a cascade of biochemical reactions succeed in achieving a particular outcome. For example, one role vitamin C plays is as a co-enzyme in the production of collagen, a protein that forms part of the structure of blood vessels, bones, cartilage and skin. In fact, the initial signs of scurvy involve the disintegration of connective tissue and blood vessels, leading to painful bleeding of the gums.

Depending on how they are classified and subdivided, there are around 14 different vitamins: A, B group (B1, 2, 3, 5, 6, 7, 9, 12), C, D, E, K1 and K2. As mentioned in the introduction, it has been proposed that flavonoids be considered vitamin P in recognition of their importance.

Vitamin A, retinol, is a fat-soluble vitamin that has antioxidant properties and is essential for the health of our eyes and immune system. Several plant carotenoids, especially alpha- and beta-carotene, are considered vitamin A precursors, also called provitamin A, from which our bodies make the vitamin. Deficiencies of vitamin A contribute to night blindness and total blindness. Being fat soluble and able to be stored in fat tissue, excessive supplementation of vitamin A may be unhealthy. Good sources of vitamin A are milk and eggs. Vitamin A precursors (alpha- and beta-carotene) are present in many plants, including basil, carrots, chillies, kale, pumpkin and sweet potato.

The vitamin B series (B1, 2, 3, 5, 6, 7, 9, 12) compounds are water soluble, so are easily excreted and require regular replenishment. The B vitamins are co-enzymes involved in a range of metabolic processes and contribute to heart, muscle and nerve health. Vitamin B1, thiamine, is required in the process that converts glucose into energy within our cells. A severe deficiency in vitamin B1 is called beriberi, which can lead to heart and muscle weakness. Good sources of vitamin B1 are the outer shell of rice (that is, in brown not white rice), some legumes such as lentils and peas, plums, Brussels sprouts, quinoa, walnuts and pork.

Vitamin B2, riboflavin, contributes to energy metabolism and healing, and may help relieve migraines (Lieberman & Bruning 2007; Lyle 2011). Deficiency symptoms of vitamin B2 include anaemia and numbness of extremities due to damaged nerves, or neuropathy (Hungerford 2012). Good sources are meat, milk, whole grains, legumes and spinach.

Vitamin B3, niacin, is also involved in the production of energy and appears to help with cholesterol levels, improving insulin sensitivity and enhancing memory (Holford 2010; Hungerford 2012). Suboptimal levels of vitamin B3 are associated with anxiety, irritability and memory problems. A severe deficiency in vitamin B3 is called pellagra, with symptoms of dementia, dermatitis and diarrhoea. Sources of vitamin B3 include legumes, meat, mushrooms, whole grains, avocado and tomatoes (Lieberman & Bruning 2007).

Vitamin B5, pantothenic acid, is a precursor to co-enzyme A. It is involved in energy, fat and neurotransmitter processes. It is most common in meat, eggs, legumes, avocados and mushrooms (Lyle 2011).

Vitamin B6, pyridoxine, is a co-enzyme involved in the health of our immune system and contributes to the balance between sodium and potassium. B6 is involved in the incorporation of iron into red blood cells. It can contribute to relieving the symptoms of insomnia and nausea (Hungerford 2012). Vitamin B6 also plays a role in the formation of the brain chemical serotonin, which contributes to the feeling of happiness, and low levels of B6 are linked to depression (Holford 2010). Good sources of B6 include eggs, meat, beans, bok choy, carrots, cashews, lentils, peas, rice and spinach.

Vitamin B7, biotin, is a co-enzyme whose deficiency can contribute to dermatitis and hair loss (Hungerford 2012). It is found in eggs, cheese, broccoli, cauliflower, legumes and sweet potatoes.

Vitamin B9, folate (the synthetic supplement form is called folic acid), is involved in maintaining amino acids, vital as the building blocks of proteins and DNA. It is a particularly important vitamin for pregnant women, because of its role in cell growth. Folate plays an important role in DNA methylation, which is a process involved in gene expression. Low levels of folate have been linked to depression (Holford 2010). Good sources of folate are meat, avocados, citrus, flax seed, kale, legumes, mustard greens, nuts, parsley, spinach and whole grains.

Vitamin B12, cobalamin, is a co-enzyme for the extraction of energy from some fats. A deficiency of B12 can cause anaemia and may also be involved in dementia (Hungerford 2012). True plants do not provide vitamin B12, although minor amounts may be available from some algae such as *Chlorella*. Good sources of vitamin B12 are meat, eggs, milk and seafood.

Vitamin C, ascorbic acid (or ascorbate) is a water-soluble strong antioxidant. Although most animals produce their own vitamin C, humans and some other primates have lost this ability, possibly due to the high amount of vitamin C provided in the plants eaten by primates and our ancestors.

Vitamin C is an antioxidant that can reduce cell and tissue damage from free radicals, and also functions as a co-enzyme to complete necessary metabolic reactions within our bodies. Vitamin C helps restore the antioxidant potential of vitamin E. The essential role of vitamin C in the production of collagen was mentioned earlier. This role has been found to be enhanced when consumed with some flavonoids, such as hesperidin and citrin in citrus and chillies (Rusznyak & Szent-Györgyi 1936). Vitamin C is damaged during cooking.

A severe deficiency of vitamin C causes scurvy, with symptoms of painful limbs, bleeding gums and lethargy. Its role in collagen production makes it important in the healing of joints, such as knees. It can relieve the symptoms of colds, reduce blood clotting, may help reduce the risk of some cancers and lower the severity of depression (Lyle 2011). Many plants are a great source of vitamin C, especially berries, citrus, capsicums, chillies and parsley. The Australian native Kakadu plum has one of the highest concentrations of vitamin C recorded.

Vitamin D is an interesting vitamin and the process of manufacturing it under our skin is similar to photosynthesising like a plant. Ultra violet sunrays hitting our skin convert a cholesterol-like compound into vitamin D. It has an important role in immunity, bone growth and hormone balance, and increases calcium and phosphorus absorption. Ricketts is a disease of severe vitamin D deficiency. Low levels of vitamin D have also been linked to the risk of dementia, eczema, muscle pain, heart problems and cancer. As well as being synthesised by exposure of our skin to sunlight, we can source vitamin D in low levels from seafood and eggs.

Vitamin E, also called alpha-tocopherol, is a fat-soluble vitamin with strong antioxidant properties that reduce damage to cells and tissue. Vitamin E travels with LDLs in our blood and appears to provide them protection from oxidative damage. It contributes to a healthy heart and immune system and may help reduce the risk of some cancers, such as prostate cancer, and of developing dementia. Plants are good sources of vitamin E, including avocados, almonds, parsley, kale and spinach.

Vitamins K1 and K2 are also fat-soluble vitamins. Vitamin K1, called phylloquinone, is produced in chloroplasts, which are structures within plant cells where photosynthesis occurs. Vitamin K1 helps reduce excessive bleeding by promoting clotting. An oversupply of vitamin K1 can interfere with the blood thinning drug warfarin. Sources of vitamin K1 include broccoli, legumes, olive oil, onions, parsley and spinach.

Vitamin K2, also known as menaquinone, is present in meat, milk, cheese and eggs. Animals convert vitamin K1 from chloroplasts in plant leaves into vitamin K2, so that grass and herb-fed animals have much more vitamin K2 than those fed corn (Lin 2018). The fermentation process also produces vitamin K2, so that natto (fermented soy) and sauerkraut (fermented cabbage) contain good levels. Vitamin K2 is essential for helping bones and teeth absorb calcium and for inhibiting calcium buildup in arteries and in kidney stones (Lin 2018).

Chapter 14
Why plants make phytochemicals

Plants are expert chemists and skilled adaptors, they make continuous self-improvements generation after generation. Consider the difference in the size of seeds on a cob of corn compared to wild grasses, from which corn originates. It is true that a cob of corn has come about because of human selection, but it was the plants that created the changes from an original wild grass seed head. People simply gave the plants the opportunity to continue their transformation, by planting preferred offspring.

The adaptability of plants has allowed them to develop a huge range of phytochemicals to help them prosper across extremes in environment. Once a seed has dispersed and germinated, plants remain rooted to the same spot for their entire lives, unless moved by floods or gardeners. They must endure whatever weather conditions are thrown at them, from heat, cold, drought and floods. Plants also have the job of dealing with herbivores and attracting flower pollinators and seed dispersers. They manufacture different phytochemicals to help them accomplish all of this.

Plants and insects have been co-evolving for a very long time. Plants are continually refining their toxins to deter insects from eating them, and insects continue to evolve to cope with the toxins. Plants are also constantly improving their chemical attractants to tempt insects and animals to pollinate their flowers and disperse their seeds.

Plants use a range of phytochemicals as signals. Eucalypt trees exude the flavonoid rutin from their roots to attract mycorrhizal fungi (Lagrange *et al.* 2001). The fungi attach to the roots, creating a crucial symbiotic relationship, helping extract soil nutrients for the tree, while the fungi receive sugars from the plant in return. Fire is a feature of many types of natural vegetation. A huge number of plants across the globe use chemicals present in the smoke from burning plant material, especially karrikinolide, to trigger or enhance seed germination (Flematti *et al.* 2004). The chemicals in smoke signal to the seeds that it is a good time to germinate while there is open space and nutrients are available in the ash. Even lettuce, a cultivated plant far removed from wild forests, has seed germination that can be enhanced by exposure to smoke (Drewes *et al.* 1995).

Plants must respond to the damaging effects of free radicals that form as an unwanted consequence of photosynthesis in chloroplasts within their leaves, and from the metabolism of energy in mitochondria within each cell. As a result of the extra source of free radicals formed during photosynthesis, plants have a greater need of antioxidants than do people and animals. Both plants and animals make the antioxidants superoxide dismutase (SOD) and glutathione. Plants also make many phytochemicals with antioxidant properties in response to free radicals, to complement SOD and glutathione, especially in times of stress such as hot, dry days (Brunetti *et al.* 2015). This role of phytochemicals in plants, complementing and enhancing the antioxidant capacity of glutathione, functions in the same way in us when we eat plants (see Chapter 4).

Phytochemicals that are important antioxidants for people include carotenoids and flavonoids. Many carotenoids, such as beta-carotene and lutein, are concentrated within the chloroplasts in plant leaves where photosynthesis occurs. These carotenoids help reduce oxidative damage to leaf cells by dealing with free radicals that are formed when photosynthesis takes place (Jaleel *et al.* 2009). Some of the same carotenoids, especially lutein, protect our eyes from oxidative damage from sunlight.

Flavonoids are found throughout plant tissues. Their concentrations fluctuate within plants in response to the plant's need for antioxidants during times of environmental stress (Close & McArthur 2002). For example, plants accumulate flavonoids, such as luteolin and quercetin, in their leaves to provide antioxidant protection from free radical damage formed under intense sunlight (Agati *et al.* 2009). Luteolin and quercetin provide antioxidant benefits to us when we consume plants. The flavonoids in tea that are so beneficial to people have a role as antioxidants in the leaves of tea plants, protecting them from free radical damage during high light intensity (Zhang *et al.* 2017).

Flavonoids play a broader role in plants than just as antioxidants. As mentioned earlier, the flavonoid rutin is exuded by roots of eucalypt trees to attract mycorrhizal fungi that help extract soil nutrients (Lagrange *et al.* 2001). The concentrations of flavonoids, such as the human health-stimulating kaempferol and myricetin, become elevated in pine leaves regrowing on trees during the initial months after a fire; this suggests that plants make flavonoids to help with healing and regeneration (Cannac *et al.* 2011).

Several flavonoids such as apigenin, kaempferol and quercetin, influence the concentrations of the plant growth hormone auxin, with high concentrations of kaempferol and quercetin associated with greater branching of flowering stalks and roots (Jansen 2002). It is tempting to speculate that these flavonoids may also influence hormones in people.

Many phytochemicals are produced in plants to deter or kill bacteria, fungi, insects and other herbivores. For example, resveratrol found in red wine protects grapes from fungal attack (Jeandet *et al.* 2014). The flavonoids in tea, especially catechins, possess antimicrobial properties that protect their leaves from diseases such as fungal blister blight (Punyasiri *et al.* 2004). Some insects take advantage of plant toxins, by concentrating them into their bodies to act as a defence against their predators, and even to attract mates (Treutter 2006).

A colourful flush of new leaf growth can be as attractive as flowers, with various shades of red, yellow and purple. These bright colours may be a warning to herbivores that the new leaves are toxic. In fact, some Australian rainforest trees contain a higher concentration of chemical defences (in the form of polyphenols) in young leaves compared to older tough leaves (Read *et al.* 2003).

The polyphenols chlorogenic acid and quercetin play a role as insect larva repellents and toxins. The tobacco army worm can cause considerable damage to peanut plants (*Arachis hypogaea*). However, wild relatives of peanuts (*Arachis kempff-mercadoi*) produce higher amounts of quercetin and chlorogenic acid, which kill a proportion of tobacco army worm larvae that feed on its leaves (Mallikarjuna *et al.* 2004). Chlorogenic acid also plays a role in repelling thrips in chrysanthemums, where it acts as a pro-oxidant, rather than antioxidant – that is, causing oxidation damage to the insects (Leiss *et al.* 2009). This role of chlorogenic acid as a free radical-like pro-oxidant is particularly interesting, because many phytochemicals provide benefits to people by working as pro-oxidants (also called electrophiles) to stimulate our cells to make the powerful antioxidant glutathione (see Chapter 4). In fact, it is thought that the stimulation of our cells by chlorogenic acid to make antioxidants such as glutathione may be an important reason why drinking coffee, which contains chlorogenic acid, benefits our cardiovascular system. It does this by reducing the oxidation of LDL 'bad' cholesterol (Butt & Sultan 2011).

Several root vegetables provide abundant health benefits. These plants include carrots, ginger, sweet potato and turmeric. Their roots store the plant's nutrients, especially over the dormant season (i.e. during winter in temperate regions and the dry season for tropical plants). To protect their precious nutrient reserves, plants produce a range of potent antimicrobial and antioxidant phytochemicals, such as gingerol in ginger and curcumin in turmeric.

Plants also make phytochemicals to attract pollinators and seed dispersers. A recent study suggests that caffeine, present in the nectar of coffee and citrus flowers, helps bees remember the location of pollen sources (Wright *et al.* 2013). Some phytochemicals, especially the anthocyanins that provide the colours of berries, may play a role in the development of memory in animals, helping them remember edible plants. Anthocyanins in blueberry skin for example, appear to have a beneficial role in memory and delaying Alzheimer's disease, and of course caffeine in coffee seeds has a brain stimulating effect (Murugaiyah & Mattson 2015).

Some scientists, such as David Kennedy of Northumbria University in England, think that a key reason we benefit so much from phytochemicals is a result of the long history of plants developing phytochemicals to stop insect herbivory and to attract insect pollinators, and subsequently seed dispersing animals. This, coupled with the insect and animal responses to those phytochemicals, has led to a vast array of fine-tuned phytochemicals and the ability of animals to cope with, and even take advantage of them (Kennedy 2014). We are the lucky beneficiaries of this long process.

Cultivation methods to enhance phytochemical production in plants

The conditions under which plants are grown affects the concentration of phytochemicals. Therefore, cultivation techniques can be refined to enhance the concentration of health-promoting phytochemicals in fruit, vegetables, herbs and spices. Plant cultivars and season of growth also influence phytochemical concentrations (Pék *et al.* 2012).

A six year trial found onions grown organically contained significantly more flavonoids and higher antioxidant capacity than conventionally grown onions (Ren *et al.* 2017). The organic method of soil management, involving crop rotation with clover and use of organic rather than synthetic fertilisers, provided the greatest phytochemical benefit. Hand weeding versus the use of herbicides and fungicides had less of an effect. A ten-year trial found that organically grown tomatoes produced with good soil organic matter contained significantly higher levels of several flavonoids, especially quercetin, than tomatoes grown conventionally with artificial fertilisers and pesticides (Mitchell *et al.* 2007).

The addition of sulphur fertilisers can increase gallic acid and sulforaphane concentration in broccoli (Pék *et al.* 2012), but using fertilisers high in nitrogen has been found to decrease sulforaphane concentration (Schonhof *et al.* 2007). In contrast, higher rates of nitrogen fertilising have been found to increase the levels of lutein and zeaxanthin in corn, though do not affect other phytochemicals such as anthocyanins and ferulic acid (Giordano *et al.* 2018). Abundant irrigation of broccoli plants reduces sulforaphane content (Pék *et al.* 2012). Increased exposure to sunlight or intense light is generally associated with increased concentrations of polyphenols, such as anthocyanins (Poiroux-Gonord *et al.* 2010).

An overall meta-analysis that reviewed the results of 343 individual studies concluded that fruit and vegetables grown organically had around 20 to 40% more antioxidant phytochemicals, especially polyphenols, than conventionally grown produce (Barański *et al.* 2014). On this basis, they calculated that organic plants provide an extra one to two serves of fruit and vegetables-worth of antioxidants and polyphenols a day, compared to conventionally grown produce.

Mycorrhizae are fungi that grow into web-like strands attached to plant roots, enhancing nutrient uptake in exchange for plant sugars. Numerous studies indicate that plants grown with mycorrhizal fungi increase their phytochemical production. For example, mycorrhizal fungi have been shown to increase polyphenols in artichokes (Ceccarelli *et al.* 2010), caffeic and rosmarinic acids in basil (Toussaint *et al.* 2007), anthocyanins and carotenoids in lettuce (Baslam *et al.* 2011) and anthocyanins in strawberries (Lingua *et al.* 2013). Mycorrhizal fungi are typically more abundant in soils high in organic matter. Therefore, it is probable that increasing soil organic matter can increase concentrations of phytochemicals in both conventional and organic agricultural crops.

Overall, it appears that pampering plants with abundant watering, pesticides and nitrogen fertilisers tends to lower the concentration of many health-promoting phytochemicals. This makes sense as many phytochemicals are produced by plants in response to insect attack and stressful growing conditions. Obviously a balanced approach in care and attention is required to produce plants that have both a high yield and good levels of phytochemicals. Growing plants in healthy soil with good organic matter and microbes such mycorrhizal fungi also tends to increase phytochemical production.

Chapter 15
Health benefits of specific fruit, vegetables, herbs and spices

Eating a wide variety of fruit and vegetables (including legumes, nuts and whole grains), and herbs and spices, plus drinking tea and coffee and eating small amounts of dark chocolate, supplies a broad range of health promoting phytochemicals. This section provides information about the phytochemicals in many beneficial plants and plant products, plausible health benefits attributed to them and scientific evidence about how they may be providing those health benefits. The 'plausible health benefits' listed for each plant are those for which, in my opinion, there is some reasonable evidence to support health claims.

Key sources of information about phytochemical, mineral and vitamin content of plants in this chapter are Food Standards of Australia and New Zealand's food nutrient database (FSANZ 2013); the United States Department of Agriculture's databases of flavonoid and nutrient contents in food (Bhagwat & Haytowitz 2015; USDA 2018); Duke (2016); Lyle (2011); Phenol Explorer (Rothwell *et al.* 2013) and PhytoHub (2017). In addition to research papers published in scientific journals, important sources of information about the health benefits of individual plants include Bharat Aggarwal and Debora Yost's (2011) book 'Healing Spices', Susanna Lyle's (2011) book 'Eat Smart Stay Well' and David Wilkinson's (2015) book 'Can Food be Medicine Against Cancer?'. Valuable sources of information about the origins and cultivation of plants are Annette McFarlane's (2010; 2011) books 'Organic Vegetable Growing' and 'Organic Fruit Growing'.

Plants do not supply preformed vitamin A, but many supply a group of carotenoids, especially alpha- and beta-carotene, which our bodies convert into vitamin A. This chapter includes information about plants with abundant provitamin A (beta-carotene equivalents) which indicates there is likely to be sufficient alpha- and beta-carotene and/or beta-cryptoxanthin present for our bodies to produce vitamin A (FSANZ 2013).

ALMONDS

Almonds are seeds from the fruit of *Prunus dulcis*, a relative of peaches and plums. The trees originate from the Mediterranean and Middle East.

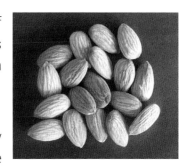

Plausible health benefits

Almonds contribute to a healthy cardiovascular system, help reduce inflammation and can lower appetite, helping with weight management. People with general nut allergies should be careful about whether to eat almonds. Almonds contain traces of cyanogenic glycosides, which are precursers to cyanide, but are safe when not eaten to excess.

Significant phytochemicals

Almonds contain the phytosterols beta-sitosterol and campesterol, the polyphenols protocatechuic and vanillic acids and flavonoids catechin, hyperin, kaempferol and quercetin. They are high in fibre, provide vitamins B1, B2, B3, B6, B9 (folate) and E, plus good amounts of calcium, magnesium and zinc.

How almonds provide health benefits

The phytochemicals in almonds, especially the flavonoids and vitamin E, provide strong antioxidant properties. A study of 60 smokers found eating 84 grams of almonds daily for four weeks significantly increased the antioxidant capacity of their blood, including enhanced production by their cells of the strong antioxidants, superoxide dismutase (SOD) and glutathione (Li *et al.*

2007). This lowered levels of oxidised fats in the blood, which is important for cardiovascular health.

The phytosterols, beta-sitosterol and campesterol, help lower the absorption of cholesterol and eating almonds has been found to improve the ratio of HDL 'good' cholesterol to LDL 'bad' cholesterol (Spiller *et al.* 1998). Almonds contain healthy monounsaturated fat, which is also thought to be good for the cardiovascular system and for relieving inflammation. The high monounsaturated fat and fibre content help fill us up, reducing the urge to over eat, therefore contribute to weight management.

APPLES

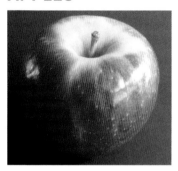

Apples are one of the most popular fruit around the globe. They grow on the deciduous tree *Malus domestica*, which originates from the Middle East and Asia (McFarlane 2011). They are relatives of apricots, peachs, plums and roses.

Plausible health benefits

Eating apples is good for digestion and general gut health, and can help lower blood pressure, therefore contributing to cardio-vascular health. Apples can also help reduce allergy symptoms. For example, children in Crete who regularly eat apples, as well as other fruit, have lower incidents of hay fever and asthma-like symptoms such as wheezing (Chatzi *et al.* 2007). They can help lower the severity of inflammatory pain, with apple cider vinegar having a particularly good reputation for relieving arthritic pain.

Significant phytochemicals

Apples contain the carotenoids beta-carotene and lutein, the phytosterols beta-sitosterol and campersterol, the poly-phenols caffeic, chlorogenic and ferulic acids, and flavonoids catechin, kaempferol and quercetin. Apples also supply large amounts of the soluble fibre pectin, and vitamins B1, B2, B3, B6, C and E. They provide minerals such as calcium, magnesium and potassium.

How apples provide health benefits

Pectin is thought to help with digestion and prevent the extremes of constipation and diarrhoea (Lyle 2011). Apples provide abundant antioxidants from the combination of vitamins C and E and various other phytochemicals, such as quercetin (Liu 2003). This can provide many benefits, including reduced damage to blood vessels and brain tissue.

The flavonoids in apples, kaempferol and quercetin, can help reduce inflammation, which can cause allergies and pain, by inhibiting the activation of NF-κB and the COX-2 enzyme. This process also thins the blood by the same mechanism as aspirin.

AVOCADOS

Avocados are the fruit of the *Persea americana* tree, originally from Mexico and Central America. They are grown in subtropical and tropical regions of the world, including eastern and south western Australia (McGuire 2016).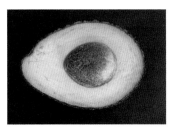
The trees are part of the Laurel family, which includes cinnamon (produced from the bark of the cinnamon tree), camphor laurels and bay leaves. Avocados are unusual in that they do not ripen until after they are picked. They are a popular addition to salads, and 'smashed avocado' is a fashionable addition to breakfast and lunch menus.

Plausible health benefits

Avocados can help with weight loss by delaying feelings of hunger. They can improve heart health by providing healthy fats, improving the ratio of HDL 'good' cholesterol to LDL 'bad' cholesterol and reducing the oxidative damage to LDLs. They can help protect our eyes from cataracts and macular degeneration. Avocados may help relieve arthritis and other painful inflammatory conditions. Laboratory trials suggest avocados could potentially contribute to inhibiting cancer development (Ding *et al.* 2007).

Significant phytochemicals

Avocados contain the carotenoids beta-carotene, lutein, violaxanthin and zeaxanthin; as well as polyphenols p-coumaric acid, minor amounts of resveratrol (the compound admired in red wine) and epigallocatechin (most abundantly found in green tea). They are one of the richest natural sources of the cholesterol-lowering beta-sitosterol (Duester 2001). Avocados are known for their healthy fat content, including the monounsaturated fat, oleic acid (which is concentrated in olive oil).

Avocados contain soluble and insoluble fibre, provitamin A, vitamins B1, B2, B3, B6, B9 (folate), C, E and K1; as well they offer a range of minerals including calcium, iodine, iron, magnesium and potassium (Dreher & Davenport 2013). They are a good source of Coenzyme Q_{10} (also called ubiquinone) and contain an unusual fat called avocatin B.

How avocados provide health benefits

In a tasty trial, people adding half an avocado to their lunch reported reduced subsequent afternoon hunger and had lower blood insulin levels for three hours following the meal, compared to those eating a similar lunch without avocados (Wien *et al.* 2013). The healthy fats in avocado will have contributed to reduced hunger. The reduction in blood insulin levels appears to be influenced by the fat content and an uncommon type of sugar found in avocados called mannoheptulose (Lyle 2011).

A separate trial involving 15 women found that those who included avocados in their diet for three weeks lowered their total cholesterol levels by an average of 8%, which was more than the 5% drop in trial participants who added complex carbohydrates rather than avocados to their diet (Colquhoun *et al.* 1992). Importantly, avocados help improve the ratio of HDL 'good' cholesterol to LDL 'bad' cholesterol. That is, they help maintain a healthy cholesterol balance (Peou *et al.* 2016; Caldas *et al.* 2017). The phytochemical beta-sitosterol, which is abundant in avocado flesh, helps achieve this balance by reducing the absorption of cholesterol from our diet and reducing the production of cholesterol by our liver (Duester 2001).

The fat content of avocados enhances the absorption of important fat-soluble phytochemicals, especially carotenoids such as beta-carotene, which our bodies convert to vitamin A. Some carotenoids in avocados, such as lutein and violaxanthin, may reduce the levels of oxidised LDLs, which are associated with atherosclerosis and heart disease. Lutein is used in the retinas of our eyes to protect them from oxidative damage and ultimately macular degeneration and cactaracts (Ribaya-Mercado & Blumberg 2004; Dreher & Davenport 2013). Eating avocados can reduce inflammation by lowering the activation of the inflammation-promoting protein NF-κB (Caldas *et al.* 2017).

Extracts of avocado have been found to promote cancer cell death in laboratory studies (Ding *et al.* 2007). A type of fat in avocados called avocatin B has been found to selectively target and destroy acute myeloid leukemia cells in a laboratory setting (Lee *et al.* 2015).

BANANAS

Bananas are the popular fruit from trees in the *Musa* genus, grown across warmer regions of the world, including eastern Australia. Flowers are grouped together under large reddish bracts. The flowers, and then ultimately the fruit, hang together at the end of a long stalk. The large banana leaves are sometimes used as plates to eat food off, in some South East Asian countries.

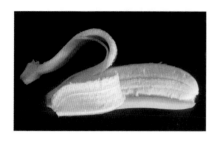

Bananas and plantains (i.e. cooking bananas) are giant herbs with succulent stems. Australia has three species of native bananas from the wet tropical rainforests of north Queensland, although one, the Daintree banana (*Musa fitzalanii*), is thought to have become extinct in the wild. The native Australian bananas retain seeds and have less flesh than cultivated varieties.

The cultivation of bananas is thought to have originated in New Guinea around 8,000 to 10,000 years ago, although may have developed concurrently in South East Asia. The varieties we commonly eat (e.g. cavendish and lady finger) are cultivars of, and hybrids between, *Musa acuminata* and *M. balbisiana*. Hybrids between these two species are sometimes called *Musa × paradisiaca*. The cultivated bananas have had their seeds greatly reduced to minute specks. Propagation of bananas is therefore by planting suckers. Natural Evolution Foods, a company developed by innovative north Queensland banana growers Krista and Robert Watkins, make banana flour which is free of gluten.

Unfortunately, the fungal disease that causes severe plant wilt, Panama disease tropical race 4, present in South East Asia, has recently been detected in a minor number of north Queensland farms. It is also present in the Northern Territory. This puts an extra strain on growers because of considerable quarantine efforts required to keep their farms disease free. Banana plants should only be sourced from reputable suppliers. There are restrictions on moving banana plants (especially to stop transport between banana biosecurity zones) with a biosecurity certificate or permit required in Australia to move banana plants (and obviously never move plants or soil from a potentially infected crop).

Plausible health benefits

Bananas may help lower blood pressure, reducing the risk of developing cardiovascular disease, including stroke. They also act as an antacid, reducing heart burn and potentially helping reduce stomach ulceration (Lyle 2011).

Significant phytochemicals

Bananas contain beta-carotene and lutein, the phytosterols campesterol and beta-sitosterol, polyphenols ferulic, gallic, p-courmaric and vanillic acids, and flavonoids catechin, kaempferol, leucocyanidin and quercetin (Vilela *et al.* 2014; Bhagwat & Haytowitz 2015; Singh *et al.* 2016). They supply vitamins B1, B2, B3, B6, B9 (folate), C and E, plus good amounts of magnesium, potassium and fibre.

How bananas provide health benefits

The potassium and fibre in bananas contribute to their capacity to help lower blood pressure and the risk of stroke. Phytosterols, for example beta-sitosterol, also play an important role in reducing blood pressure (Choudhary & Tran 2011). In addition, beta-sitosterol helps reduce the absorption of cholesterol from our diet and lower the production of cholesterol by our liver, leading to healthy cholesterol levels (Duester 2001).

Bananas, especially slightly unripe ones, seem to provide relief from heart burn and possibly stomach ulcers, by promoting the production of mucous lining of the stomach (Best *et al.* 1984). A laboratory experiment fed a group of rats leucocyanidin, a flavonoid extracted from plantain bananas, prior to giving them aspirin. Another group of rats was given aspirin without prior feeding with leucocyanidin. Rats fed leucocyanidin extracted from plantain bananas developed significantly fewer stomach ulcers from the aspirin compared to the other rats (Lewis *et al.* 1999).

BASIL

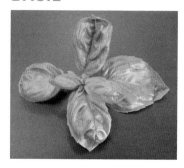

Basil (*Ocimum basilicum*, also called sweet basil) is a herb of the mint family, Lamiaceae. Its crushed leaves give off a strong aroma and it is a favourite ingredient in Italian recipes, such as pesto, as well as being widely used in Thai and Vietnamese cooking (including different basil varieties). It was once said that a man should give basil to a woman to attract her affections; and young ladies should put basil on the windowsill to indicate that a suitor was welcome (Shipard 2003; Aggarwal 2010).

Plausible health benefits

There are many afflictions thought to be helped by basil. Its roles in these include wound healing, and relief from colds, diabetes, inflammatory pain, acne, gout and headaches (Shipard 2003; Aggarwal 2010).

Significant phytochemicals

Basil contains very high levels of beta-carotene, as well as beta-ocimene, limonene, lycopene and menthol. It provides the polyphenols caffeic and rosmarinic acids and quercetin. Caffeic and rosmarinic acid concentrations can be increased in basil plants grown with symbiotic mycorrhizal soil fungi (Toussaint *et al.* 2007). Basil also contains provitamin A, vitamins B1, B2, B6, C and E; and the minerals magnesium, phosphorus, potassium, selenium and zinc.

How basil provides health benefits

Phytochemicals in basil, especially rosmarinic acid, provide strong antioxidant benefits. Basil phytochemicals can inhibit the actions of the inflammation-causing protein NF-kB, which may help relieve inflammatory pain (Aggarwal & Shishodia 2004; Lyle

2011). Lyle (2011) recommends using basil for its antimicrobial benefits to treat skin infections, by mixing basil in diluted eucalyptus oil to apply externally.

BEETROOT

Beetroot is the large, red bulb of the Mediterranean herb *Beta vulgaris*. The leaves can also be eaten. Sugarbeet is another variety of *Beta vulgaris*, sometimes used to produce sugar (sucrose). Beetroots are in the Chenopodiaceae family, which includes quinoa and spinach.

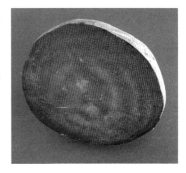

Plausible health benefits

Beetroots and beetroot juice are valued for contributing to cardiovascular health, especially by helping reduce the oxidative damage to LDL 'bad' cholesterol and lowering blood pressure. The reduced blood pressure and associated improvement in blood flow has given beetroot a reputation for improving exercise performance. Beetroot juice can help relieve the pain of osteoarthritis.

Significant phytochemicals

Beetroots contain betanin, a type of betalain which are nitrogen-containing phytochemicals that provide the red colouring. Beetroots also contain beta-carotene and small amounts of the flavonoids luteolein and quercetin. Beetroots provide high levels of nitrate, >250 mg per 100 grams (Ormsbee *et al.* 2013). They also have moderately high folate (vitamin B9) concentrations, as well as smaller quantities of vitamins B1, B2, B3, B6, C and E. Beetroots provide minerals including calcium, iron and magnesium.

How beetroots provide health benefits

The nitrate in beetroots is converted in our body into nitrite then onto nitric oxide. Betanin probably also contributes to promoting nitric oxide (Esatbeyoglu *et al.* 2015). Nitric oxide relaxes blood vessel muscles, lowering blood pressure. This leads to better blood flow, which promotes better cardiovascular health. Human trials show that drinking beetroot juice, or eating baked beetroots, can improve exercise performance, such as cycling and running, and helps with post-exercise muscle recovery. This effect comes primarily through the benefits of enhanced nitric oxide (Ormsbee *et al.* 2013).

Betanin also provides strong antioxidant benefits, including promoting glutathione production (Butera *et al.* 2002). These anti-oxidant effects can protect LDL 'bad' cholesterol from oxidative damage (Butera *et al.* 2002; Esatbeyoglu *et al.* 2015). Betanin also reduces inflammation by inhibiting the inflammatory enzyme COX-2 (Esatbeyoglu *et al.* 2015). As a result, consuming betanin-rich beetroot juice has been found to lower the pain of osteoarthritis (Pietrzkowski *et al.* 2010). Its anti-inflammatory properties probably contribute to reducing muscle soreness after intense exercise.

BLUEBERRIES

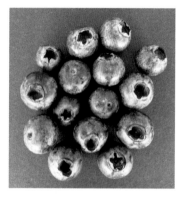

Blueberries (various species and hybrid cultivars of *Vaccinium*, including *Vaccinium angustifolium*, *Vaccinium ashei*, *Vaccinium australe* and *Vaccinium corymbosum*) are the blue/purple berries of small shrubs related to Azaleas and Rhododendrons (McFarlane 2011).

Plausible health benefits
Consumption of blueberries may boost mental performance in children and adults, and may slow the development of cognitive decline in older adults (Devore *et al.* 2012). Blueberries contribute to cardiovascular health and can reduce inflammation.

Significant phytochemicals

Blueberries contain high levels of a range of anthocyanins, including cyanidin, delphinidin, malvidin, peonidin and petunidin (Bhagwat & Haytowitz 2015). These anthocyanins provide the dark blue colour of the fruit. Blueberries also contain other flavonoids kaempferol, myricetin and quercetin, vitamins B1, B2, B6, B9 (folate), C and E, plus magnesium, phosphorus and potassium.

How blueberries provide health benefits

People drinking wild blueberry juice daily for 12 weeks have been found to improve aspects of their memory (Krikorian *et al.* 2010). A recent UK study involving 21 children aged 7 to 10, found that they improved in several mental tests, including word recall and recognition, within several hours of drinking wild blueberry drinks. The drinks provided the equivalent of eating 120 grams of wild blueberries, and even better results occurred when drinking the equivalent of 240 grams of blueberries (Whyte *et al.* 2016). The antioxidant and anti-inflammatory effects of the range of polyphenols, including anthocyanins, present in blueberries are thought to have provided this benefit. The researchers also suggested anthocyanins increase brain cell signalling. In particular, there is evidence that flavonoids, especially anthocyanins in blueberries, can promote or maintain levels of a protein found in the brain called brain derived neurotrophic factor (BDNF). This protein enhances the growth and survival of brain neurones and has an important role in learning and memory (Whyte *et al.* 2016). There also appears to be an association between low BDNF levels and abundant beta-amyloid, the peptide associated with Alzheimer's disease.

A trial involving 30 adults with metabolic syndrome found that taking blueberry extracts for six months had several positive effects. It reduced their levels of uric acid, lowered indicators of DNA and lipoprotein oxidation (that is, reduced damage to LDL 'bad' cholesterol), lessened injury to blood vessel cell membranes and reduced C-reactive protein levels, which are an indicator of inflammation (Pastor *et al.* 2016). The antioxidant and anti-inflammatory effects of the anthocyanins in blueberries, which reduce oxidation of LDLs, help reduce the risk of cardiovascular diseases (Chen *et al.* 2006). Another study involving 18 men confirmed drinking wild blueberry juice reduces DNA oxidation (Riso *et al.* 2013).

Blueberries can reduce glucose absorption into the blood by inhibiting the release of a digestive enzyme called alpha-glucosidase, which is produced in the lining of the small intestine (McDougall *et al.* 2005). This can help with weight management.

BROCCOLI AND CAULIFLOWERS

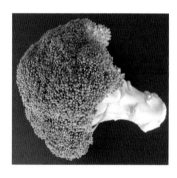

Broccoli and cauliflowers are the immature flowering heads of different cultivars of *Brassica oleracea* var. *botrytis*, which originate from the Mediterranean (McFarlane 2010). They are typically steamed or cooked briefly. It is important not to cook them for too long, that is not for more than a few minutes, because the heat damages an enzyme called myrosinase. When broccoli and cauliflower cells are broken by cutting or chewing, myrosinase mixes with the inert phytochemicals glucobrassicin and glucoraphanin and converts them into their healthy active forms indole-3-carbinol (I3C) and sulforaphane. Damaging myrosinase by cooking for more than a few minutes reduces the amount of I3C and sulforaphane activated.

Plausible health benefits

Broccoli and cauliflowers are particularly healthy plants to eat on a regular basis. They help stimulate the removal of toxins from our system, and provide antioxidant and anti-inflammatory benefits that contribute to reducing the risk of developing many chronic diseases, such as some cancers, cardiovascular disease and dementia.

Significant phytochemicals

In addition to the sulphur compounds I3C and sulforaphane, broccoli and cauliflower contain beta-carotene, the phytosterols beta-sitosterol, brassicasterol and campesterol, and polyphenols caffeic acid and flavonoids kaempferol, myricetin and quercetin (PhytoHub; Bhagwat & Haytowitz 2015). They also supply provitamin A, vitamins B1, B2, B3, B6, B9 (folate), C (in high amounts) and E, with minerals calcium, magnesium and good amounts of potassium.

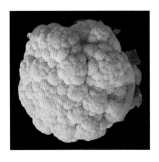

How broccoli and cauliflower provide health benefits

Chinese trials show that drinking broccoli shoot extracts increases the excretion of air pollutants, such as benzene, through urine (Kensler et al. 2011; Egner et al. 2014). The researchers considered sulforaphane responsible for enhancing the detoxification process. Sulforaphane activates the protein Nrf2, which stimulates the body's production of the antioxidant glutathione which is also involved in detoxification by promoting the production of phase 2 detoxifying enzymes (Surh 2011; Gupta et al. 2014).

Daily consumption of sulforaphane capsules produced from broccoli sprouts has been found to help reduce irritability and improve social interactions. This was determined in a trial involving 22 young men with autism spectrum disorder and a history of behavioural problems (Singh et al. 2014). Sulforaphane's capacity to stimulate the body's antioxidant glutathione and contribute to the removal of toxins, was thought to be the explanation of these benefits.

Sulforaphane and I3C have been shown in laboratory experiments of cultured cells and rodent studies to stop cancer cells multiplying, to inhibit the growth of new blood vessels around tumours and to promote the death of cancer cells (Wilkinson 2015).

BRUSSELS SPROUTS AND CABBAGES

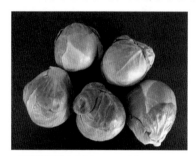

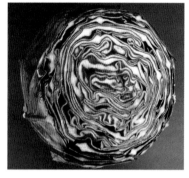

Brussels sprouts are the engorged leaf buds of *Brassica gemmifera*, originating in western Europe. The younger, smaller sprouts provide the best flavour (McFarlane 2010). Cabbages (*Brassica oleracea* var. *capitata*) are one of the oldest cultivated vegetables. With their ability to be eaten raw, in soups and fermented in sauerkraut, they were a central player in European vegetable gardens of the Middle Ages (Bloch-Dano & Fagan 2012). These days, Brussels sprouts are usually steamed or cooked briefly. Similar to broccoli, cooking Brussels sprouts or cabbage for too long - for more than a few minutes, damages the enzyme myrosinase. This enzyme is critical for converting inert phytochemicals to their healthy active forms, I3C and sulforaphane, when the plant is cut or chewed.

Plausible health benefits
Brussels sprouts and cabbages can reduce inflammation, contributing to healthy brain function, and may inhibit the development of some cancers. They can stimulate the removal of

toxins from our bodies.

Significant phytochemicals

Like many plants in their family, Brussels sprouts and cabbages contain the sulphur compounds indole-3-carbinol (I3C) and sulforaphane. They also supply beta-carotene, the phytosterols brassicasterol, campesterol, and beta-sitosterol, and the flavonoids apigenin, luteolin, naringinen (also common in grapefruit), kaempferol and good amounts of quercetin (PhytoHub; Bhagwat & Haytowitz 2015). They contain provitamin A, vitamins B1, B2, B3, B6, B9 (folate), C and E, with minerals calcium, magnesium and good amounts of potassium.

How Brussels sprouts and cabbages provide health benefits

The flavonoids provide important antioxidant and anti-inflammatory benefits. Most of the research into plants in the cabbage family have focused on I3C and sulforaphane. Both of these sulphur compounds activate the protein Nrf2, which triggers the production of powerful antioxidants within our cells (glutathione and SOD). Sulforaphane can reach the brain, providing direct antioxidant benefits and reduced oxidation of brain tissue (Corbi *et al.* 2016). Sulforaphane can also help increase the number of mitochondria (the energy processing plants within cells), helping burn more energy (Nagata *et al.* 2017).

Brussels sprouts and cabbages are valuable plants in the fight to prevent cancer development. As described earlier for broccoli and cauliflowers, I3C (abundant in Brussels sprouts) and sulforaphane have been shown in laboratory experiments of cultured cells and rodent studies to help prevent the development, survival and spread of some cancer cells (Wilkinson 2015).

CAPSICUMS AND CHILLIES (BELL PEPPERS)

There is a huge variety of capsicums and chillies, all of which are species and varieties of *Capsicum*. Some botanists consider all capsicums and chillies to be varieties of the one species, *Capsicum annum*. Others consider *Capsicum annum* to specifically describe capsicums, with chillies thought of as distinct species, for example the bird's eye chilli, 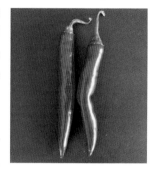 *Capsicum frutescens*. All originate from Central and South America. The name 'bell peppers' reflects the association Christopher Columbus made between these pungent fruit and the highly valuable black pepper of the spice trade, which originated in India.

Plausible health benefits

Capsicums and chillies can help reduce pain and inflammation, such as arthritis. They may be of benefit in helping to reduce the chance of developing blood clots, heart disease, type 2 diabetes and some cancers. They can also help in weight loss (Aggarwal & Yost 2011). Excessive consumption of chillies has been linked with stomach ulcers (Lyle 2011). Capsicums and chillies contain lectins, which can promote inflammation in some people, who may be better off avoiding capsicums and chillies. Cooking degrades a proportion of their lectins.

Significant phytochemicals

Capsicums and chillies contain a group of alkaloids called capsaicinoids. The various capsaicinoids are responsible for the heat of chillies, especially capsaicin. More than acting simply as a deterrant to animals, it seems possible that capsaicinoids evolved as protection against fungal attack of the seeds (Tewksbury *et al.* 2008). Self-defence 'pepper sprays' contain capsaicinoids, wreaking particular havoc if sprayed into someone's eyes. The degree of heat in chillies varies with the concentration of capsaicin and is measured using the Scoville scale. Capsaicinoids are soluble in fats and oils, not water, therefore drinking water does not quench the chilli heat, but milk will help because of the fat it contains.

Capsicums and chillies also contain the carotenoids alpha- and beta-carotene and lutein, and the flavonoids hersperidin, luteolin and myrcetin. They have quite high levels of vitamin C (around 200 mg per 100 grams, compared to about 55 mg per 100 grams of oranges). They also contain provitamin A, vitamins B1, B2, B3, B6, B9 (folate), E and K1, plus calcium and magnesium.

How capsicums and chillies provide health benefits

Capsaicinoids bind to receptors in our mouth creating the heat sensation, and over time the density of receptors reduces, allowing a chilli enthusiast to eat hotter and hotter chillies (Brunning 2015). Birds do not seem to have the receptors for capsaicinoids, and therefore can be seen happily gorging on hot chillies with no apparent suffering. In response to capsaicinoids, receptors send messages to the brain that can activate the release of various compounds, including the blood vessel dilator bradykinin. Chillies also cause the release of endorphins, which can block the actions of compounds involved in the transmission of pain signals, such as Substance P. This is probably key to reductions in the perception of pain, including arthritis, that people can experience when eating chillies.

Lutein, beta-carotene, flavonoids and the high levels of vitamin C provide good antioxidant benefits, including protecting our eyes, brain tissue and blood vessels from oxidative damage.

CHERRIES

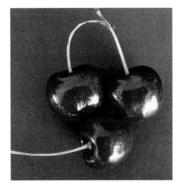

Cherries are the bright red, sweet fruit of the *Prunus avium* tree, which originates in Europe and western Asia (McFarlane 2010). They are close relatives of nectarines and peaches.

Plausible health benefits

Cherries help reduce inflammatory pain, such as gout and post exercise muscle soreness. They also contribute to healthy blood vessels and a good memory (Lyle 2011).

Significant phytochemicals

Cherries contain beta-carotene, the anthocyanins cyanidin and peonidin, and other flavonoids isorhamnetin, kaempferol and quercetin (Bhagwat & Haytowitz 2015). Cherries supply vitamins B1, B2, B3, B6, B9 (folate), C and a small amount of vitamin E. They have a range of minerals, including calcium, a good amount of iodine, magnesium and potassium.

How cherries provide health benefits

Cherries provide strong antioxidant and anti-inflammatory benefits, helping relieve the aches and pains that can follow strenuous exercise. For example, a study of 16 cyclists found that drinking cherry extracts reduced indictors of oxidative stress (lipid hydroperoxides) and inflammation (C-reactive protein) in their blood following repeated, high intensity cycling (Bell *et al.* 2014). A reduction in inflammation markers (inter-leukin-6, C-reactive protein and uric acid) was also found when marathon runners drank a cherry extract before and for two days after a marathon (Howatson *et al.* 2010). By reducing uric acid levels, cherries contribute to lowering the incidence or severity of the painful inflammation condition, gout. Their antioxidant and anti-inflammatory capacity will also help with cardiovascular health.

CHOCOLATE (COCOA AND DARK CHOCOLATE)

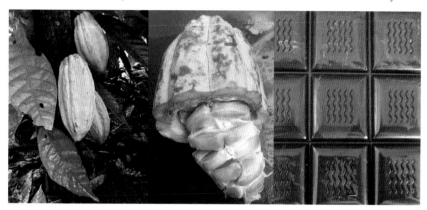

Most people will appreciate the scientific name of the cacao tree which provides us with chocolate: *Theobroma cacao* - which means 'food of the gods'. Chocolate is made from the seeds that develop within large yellow pods. The tree grows naturally in the rainforests of the Amazon and Central America, where chocolate has been consumed (mostly as a drink) by South and Central American people for thousands of years. It is now grown across many tropical regions of the world, including the Tully to Mossman region of north eastern Australia, with a collection of growers contributing to Charley's Chocolate Factory and Daintree Estates. A 100% dark chocolate cocoa mass with no added sugar is one of many chocolates produced by Stevo's Super Chocolate at Yungaburra in north Queensland. By making cocoa butter from their cocoa pods, Stevo's produce a range of chocolates made from 100% Australian ingredients.

Plausible health benefits

The most celebrated benefit of chocolate is, of course, its ability to make us feel happy. It also provides benefits to our circulation. Associated with this are boosts to brain function and memory (reducing the risk or impact of dementia), a reduction in the oxidation damage of LDL 'bad' cholesterol and lowering of blood pressure. Regular consumption of dark chocolate, with around 70% or more cocoa, appears to help reduce the risk of developing type 2 diabetes, heart disease and stroke. These benefits are less likely to come from chocolates with lower percentages of cocoa and higher sugar content than are found in dark chocolate.

Significant phytochemicals

There are a wide range of health-promoting phytochemicals found in dark chocolate. These include the polyphenols caffeic and p-coumaric acids, resveratrol (also found in red wine) and flavonoids catechins (abundant in tea) and quercetin. Good quality, dark chocolate can provide beta-carotene and vitamins B1, B2, B6 and E. It contains minerals such as calcium, iodine, iron, magnesium, phosphorus, potassium and zinc.

The popular mentally stimulating alkaloids, caffeine and theobromine, are also found in chocolate. While they are toxic at high concentrations, it is unlikely there has ever been a documented case of 'death by chocolate' and you would probably have to gorge on a lot of chocolate for it to do serious harm (Adamafio 2013). Milk and especially white chocolate are lower in theobromine; however, a big feed of dark chocolate can cause some harmful effects, such as agitation, insomnia and even nausea. Toxic effects of chocolate are known in dogs and horses. The reason chocolate is lethal to dogs is thought to be because they break down theobromine more slowly than humans do. Combined with their lower body weight compared to us, this leads quickly to poisoning (Adamafio 2013; Brunning 2015).

How chocolate provides health benefits

The Kuna people, who live on an island off the coast of Panama, are the celebrities of research into links between chocolate consumption and heart health. They traditionally drink a lot of minimally processed chocolate. A recent study has found that Kuna people living on islands have better health, especially lower blood pressure, than their relatives who have moved to Panama City. The island Kuna people drink around ten times more minimally processed chocolate, and eat around four times the amount of fish and twice as much fruit as their urban relatives (McCullough *et al.* 2006). The chocolate they drink is high in flavonoids, especially catechins, which is thought to provide vascular benefits.

Dark chocolate has been shown to reduce oxidative damage to LDL 'bad' cholesterol and to increase the relative amount of HDL 'good' cholesterol, an effect attributed to its flavonoid content (Wan *et al.* 2001; Mursu *et al.* 2004). The flavonoids in dark chocolate provide further heart benefits by limiting aggregation of blood platelets, that is thinning the blood, in a similar way to aspirin. They can also increase blood flow and lower blood pressure by enhancing nitric oxide availability, which relaxes blood vessel muscles (Pearson *et al.* 2002). For example, a study involving 45 healthy adults found eating dark chocolate, or drinking sugar-free cocoa, increased blood flow and reduced blood pressure, as a result of increased nitric oxide production in blood vessels (Faridi *et al.* 2008).

The improved blood circulation provided by dark chocolate has many flow-on benefits. A study of 42 scuba divers found that the half of participants who ate 30 grams of dark chocolate 90 minutes before a dive showed improved blood vessel dilation. This improvement was associated with increased levels of nitric oxide in their blood, reducing the stress of diving on their circulatory system (Theunissen *et al.* 2015).

A study involving 20 people with high blood pressure found that eating dark chocolate not only reduces blood pressure but can also improve insulin sensitivity (Grassi *et al.* 2005). It is worth noting that highly processed white or milk chocolate does not provide the same improvements in blood pressure and insulin sensitivity as dark chocolate because it has extra sugar and fewer phytochemicals.

A trial involving 90 people with memory impairment found that consuming beverages containing chocolate flavonoids daily for eight weeks improved mental performance (Desideri *et al.* 2012). That is, participants consuming a drink with abundant chocolate flavonoids improved their scores on mental tests to a greater degree than participants who drank an extract with a low concentration of chocolate flavonoids. The researchers thought that the improved performance may be due to the chocolate flavonoids improving blood flow and improving insulin removal from the blood system. High insulin levels have been linked to cognitive decline (Desideri *et al.* 2012).

Some dark chocolate may contain trace amounts of the alkaloid theophylline, which is also found in tea. Theophylline opens the airways within the lungs to make breathing easier (Sharangi 2009). Caffeine, which is chemically very similar to the bronchodilator theophylline, can also increase lung capacity and ease of breathing to some extent (Welsh *et al.* 2010).

Chocolate can contribute to gut health. A study involving 20 people found that drinking a chocolate extract with high levels of flavonoids increased the growth of beneficial gut bacteria, *Bifidobacterium* spp. and *Lactobacillus* spp. (Tzounis *et al.* 2011).

It is not yet clear how chocolate makes us feel happy, but it most likely involves several complementary factors. Chocolate contains the amino acids phenylethylamine and tyrosine, which can improve mood by promoting the neurotransmitter dopamine. Modified versions of phenylethylamine are used in some antidepressant drugs. Chocolate probably also makes us feel good by stimulating the release of another neurotransmitter, serotonin. The improvement in blood flow in our brain could contribute to enhanced mood, as could the stimulating effects of caffeine and theobromine. Perhaps, chocolate also gives us pleasure by simply being delicious.

CITRUS

Citrus are some of our most popu-lar fruit. Citrus include oranges (*Citrus sinensis*), lemons (*Citrus limon*), limes (*Citrus aurantiifolia*) and mandarins (*Citrus reticulata*). Grapefruit, *Citrus X paradisi*, described separately, is a large citrus fruit which is a cross between an orange and a pomelo. Australia has several native citrus, including

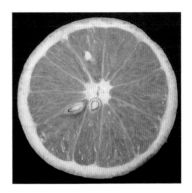

finger limes (*Citrus australasica*), which are discussed with other bush food in Chapter 16.

Citrus originate from many localities across the Middle East, Asia, through to Australia. The large, juicy fruits we enjoy today have been improved by thousands of years of plant selection. Citrus hold a special place in the history of nutritional research. Scurvy was the curse of long expedi-tions, especially at sea, causing a huge toll on sailors. In 1747, the British Royal Navy surgeon, James Lind, undertook a trial of treatments that were considered possible scurvy cures at the time. One treatment involved sailors drinking sea water, another dilute sulphuric acid. The successful treatment required sailors to eat oranges and lemons. Eventually this led to the British Navy incorporating citrus into the diet of sailors. When the navy began using limes, which were more easily sourced than oranges or lemons, the British sailors gained the nickname 'Limeys'. Unfortunately, limes contain considerably less vitamin C than oranges and lemons, and therefore didn't provide the level of scurvy protection that other citrus can.

Plausible health benefits

Citrus fruits, especially oranges and lemons, successfully prevent and treat scurvy, the disease caused by severe vitamin C deficiency. Citrus can improve mental alertness and probably reduce the duration and symptoms of hay fever-related allergies and a cold. Citrus can contribute to a healthy cardiovascular system, with lemons in particular said to strengthen blood vessels (Woodward 2014). There is some initial laboratory evidence that citrus may provide a valuable contribution to reducing the risk of developing some cancers.

Significant phytochemicals

The citrus smell of oranges and lemons is due to an oil called limonene. Citrus contain beta-carotene, citric acid and the flavonoids apigenin, hesperetin, kaempferol, luteolin, naringenin, quercetin and tangeretin. The highest concentration of some phytochemicals, especially limonene and tangeretin, are found in the peel and white pith of citrus, making the consumption of some rind and pith beneficial. Pectin, which is an important fibre, is also found in the pith and rind. Citrus contain good levels of vitamin C, and also contain vitamins B1, B2, B3, B6 and E. They provide minerals including calcium, iodine, iron, magnesium, phosphorus, potassium and zinc.

How citrus provide health benefits

Citrus prevent and treat scurvy because the vitamin C they contain is a co-enzyme required in the production of collagen, a protein that forms part of blood vessels, bones, cartilage in joints, and skin. In the initial signs of scurvy, connective tissue and blood vessels start to disintegrate leading to pain and bleeding gums. Eating citrus heals scurvy.

In addition to vitamin C, the flavonoids hesperetin, kaempferol, naringenin and quercetin in citrus provide powerful antioxidant benefits. These antioxidants can reduce or inhibit damage to cell membranes, proteins and arteries. Flavonoids, especially hesperetin, which is abundant in citrus, have been shown to limit inflammation, through their ability to inhibit over-expression of the protein COX-2. They also help lower allergic reactions by reducing the release of histamine (Tsujiyama *et al.* 2013).

A UK study involving 24 men found that drinking orange juice containing flavonoids, especially hesperetin, and added orange fibre, improved mental alertness (Alharbi *et al.* 2016). The flavonoid tangeretin (concentrated in citrus peel) may be beneficial in helping to reduce nerve damage associated with Parkinson's disease (Vauzour *et al.* 2010).

Several phytochemicals in citrus have shown potential to contribute to the protection against cancer. Naringenin can help fight cancer growth by inhibiting the activation of the inflammatory protein NF-kB and vascular endothelial growth factor (VEGF), while promoting cancer cell death (Li *et al.* 2017). Tangeretin has been shown to activate the protein p53, promoting the death of cancer cells in laboratory experiments, and to reduce NF-kB levels in breast cancer tissue in rat studies (Dong *et al.* 2014; Gul *et al.* 2017). The oil limonene stimulates the detoxification process, and has been shown in laboratory experiments to have anticancer properties (Miller *et al.* 2011). Limonene has been demonstrated to be absorbed into breast tissue, where it may help reduce the chance of developing cancer.

COFFEE

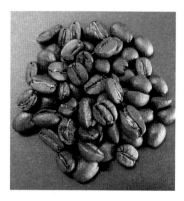

Coffee is a brew made from roasted seeds of the north African trees *Coffea arabica* (arabica coffee) and *Coffea canephora* (robusta coffee). Arabica coffee beans are usually considered the better tasting. Coffee trees are now grown in tropical and subtropical regions around the world, especially in Australia, Brazil, Ethiopia, New Guinea and South East Asia. Coffee seeds germinate easily and abundantly, and when spread by birds, are able to establish under dense forest canopies. This has caused it to become a problematic weed in some rainforests of the wet tropics of northern Australia. Where practical, especially in small orchards, netting coffee trees can help stop birds eating and spreading seeds (Webster 2017).

Plausible health benefits

The most obvious effect of coffee is its ability to stimulate attention and possibly maintain memory. Regular consumption of coffee has also been linked to reduced incidence of Parkinson's disease, Alzheimer's disease and some cancers (e.g. stomach), plus better liver health. Coffee drinking may help maintain cardiovascular health and contribute slightly to weight loss. Some asthmatics may find that after drinking coffee, they are temporarily able to breathe more easily.

Excessive consumption of coffee can cause nausea, headaches and inability to sleep. Coffee seems to be mildly addictive, sometimes causing cravings and headaches in its absence.

Significant phytochemicals

Coffee is a primary source of the alkaloid caffeine, and it also contains some theobromine (the main alkaloid in chocolate). It has the polyphenols caffeic, chlorogenic, ferulic and P-coumaric acids and flavonoids catechin and myricetin. Coffee contains vitamins B1, B2, B3, B6, B9 (folate) and E. It provides minor amounts of the minerals calcium, iron, magnesium, potassium, phosphate, selenium and zinc.

How coffee provides health benefits

The alkaloid caffeine is the ingredient that enables coffee to improve mental alertness. Caffeine blocks the neurotransmitter adenosine from attaching to brain cell receptors. Adenosine makes us feel drowsy, and by blocking adenosine's access to brain cells, caffeine keeps us alert (Brunning 2015). Caffeine also increases the availability or responsiveness of dopamine receptors, allowing more dopamine to communicate feelings of pleasure and reward (Volkow *et al.* 2015).

A Costa Rican study found some evidence that drinking several cups of coffee daily improved heart health in people who rapidly metabolise caffeine, but increased the risk of heart attack in people who metabolise caffeine slowly (Cornelis *et al.* 2006). Polyphenols in coffee, including chlorogenic acid, provide antioxidant benefits and can reduce the oxidation of LDL 'bad' cholesterol, which may account for some observed cardiovascular health benefits (Butt & Sultan 2011). Recent research suggests coffee may enhance the efficiency of energy production by mitochondria in heart cells (Ale-Agha *et al.* 2018).

Coffee stimulates metabolism, and therefore may help muscles burn fat, and this is likely to help with weight loss, but to a limited degree. Caffeine is metabolised in our bodies over many hours, with half of the caffeine ingested typically broken down within five hours, but taking up to 30 hours in some people (Crozier *et al.* 2012). The Costa Rican study mentioned above compared people who had different genetic versions of an enzyme (CYP1A2) that leads to either fast or slow caffeine metabolism. Those with slow caffeine metabolism, who break down caffeine slowly, showed some increased risk of heart attack after two, and especially after four or more, cups of coffee daily. This is possibly due to the role of caffeine in blocking adenosine receptors, because adenosine contributes to blood vessel dilation (Cornelis *et al.* 2006). Therefore, slow removal of caffeine from the blood stream could limit the dilation of blood vessels and increase blood pressure.

Recently, a Californian court is reported to have ruled that coffee suppliers should warn consumers that coffee contains acrylamide (Hsu 2018). Acrylamide is a compound that can form during the coffee bean roasting process. It can also form during frying of many plant products including potatoes and toasting bread (Mucci & Wilson 2008). Acrylamide has been found to be carcinogenic (that is it can cause cancer) in some animal tests and is listed as group 2A carcinogen for humans, meaning it is a probable carcinogen (Virk-Baker *et al.* 2014). However, the amount of acrylamide typically consumed in coffee is small. A review of human studies has found no clear evidence that consuming food containing acrylamide is linked to the rate of developing a range of cancers, and further research is needed to determine the amount of acrylamide that is dangerous to people (Mucci & Wilson 2008; Virk-Baker *et al.* 2014).

A review of seven human trials concluded that drinking one or two cups of coffee can modestly improve the ease of breathing and lung function for several hours (Welsh *et al.* 2010). This appears to be due to the effect of caffeine, which is chemically very similar to the bronchodilator theophylline, in opening the airways in lungs. The authors of that study warned that drinking coffee prior to lung function tests could over-state the strength of lungs, hindering appropriate diagnosis and medication for lung problems, such as asthma.

Caffeine can increase insulin resistance by reducing the amount of glucose absorbed in muscles (Cano-Marquina *et al*. 2013). However, the polyphenols in coffee appear to counter this effect by slowing the rate of glucose absorption from the gut and increasing glucose absorption from the blood into cells (de Mejia & Ramirez-Mares 2014). Reviews of multiple coffee studies have concluded that overall, drinking coffee without added sugar helps reduce the chance of developing type 2 diabetes (Huxley *et al*. 2009; Grosso *et al*. 2017).

CORN (MAIZE)

Corn is the large seed head of the *Zea mays* grass, originating from Mexico and Central America. It is a type of grain thought to have been bred in Mexico thousands of years ago from a wild grass called teosinte (McGuire 2016). Corn seeds come in a variety of colours, but the most common cobs of corn have yellow seeds. Australian researcher, Tim O'Hare, has crossed a 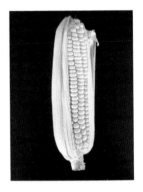 purple variety with yellow sweet corn to produce a purple sweet corn, high in anthocyanins. The word corn originally referred to any seed, with maize being the name for *Zea mays*. However, the names corn and maize are now both used to refer to *Zea mays*.

Plausible health benefits

Eating corn can help protect our eyes from cataracts and macular degeneration. Corn provides antioxidant and anti-in-flammatory benefits and may contribute to reducing the risk of developing some cancers and cardiovascular disease.

Significant phytochemicals

Corn contains good levels of several carotenoids, including beta-carotene, lutein and zeaxanthin, the phytosterols beta-sit-osterol and campesterol, and anthocyanins plus ferulic acid

(Luo & Wang 2012; Duke 2016). Corn also provides vitamins B1, B3, B6, B9 (folate), C and E, and minerals including magnesium and selenium.

How corn provides health benefits

Lutein and zeaxanthin, abundant in corn, are essential antioxidants that help protect our eyes from cataracts and macular degeneration. Anthocyanins and ferulic acid in corn are thought to help inhibit the development of tumours, primarily through their anti-inflammatory properties (Luo & Wang 2012). The phytosterols, beta-sitosterol and campesterol, inhibit the absorption of cholesterol from food, and combined with the antioxidant properties from anthocyanins and ferulic acid, may help reduce the risk of cardiovascular disease.

FLAX SEED (LINSEED)

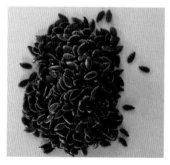

The seeds of the flax plant *Linum usitatissimum*, are also known as linseed. The flax plant is an attractive blue-flowered herb that originates from the Middle East and western Mediterranean region. It has been cultivated for thousands of years as a multiple-purpose plant providing food, oil and fibre (linen). Flax seed is probably one the healthiest seeds available.

Plausible health benefits

Flax seed contributes to cardiovascular health by reducing blood clotting and inflammation, and lowering LDL 'bad' cholesterol levels. It helps relieve inflammatory diseases such as arthritis, improves mood and reduces the chance of developing dementia.

Flax seed, especially the husk, contains minor traces of cyanogenic glycosides, which are precursers to cyanide. They are also found in the seeds of several plants including apples, almonds and peaches. Therefore, pregnant and breast-feeding women should not eat flax seed, nor should very young children, and nobody should consume huge amounts (e.g. more than about 60 to 100 grams) of raw husked flax seed at a time (Castleman 2017; Lyle 2011).

Significant phytochemicals

Flax seed has a high concentration of phytosterols, especially beta-sitosterol and campesterol. Flax seed are one of the best sources of polyphenol compounds called lignans, especially secoisolariciresinol, and they also contain p-couramic acid. They are abundant in the omega 3 fat, alpha-linolenic acid (ALA) and fibre. They provide vitamins, especially B1 and E, and the minerals calcium, manganese, selenium and zinc (Lyle 2011).

How flax seed provide health benefits

A good proportion of the omega 3 fat, ALA, in flax seed enters our blood stream. ALA in flax seed reduces inflammation because it is one of the building blocks of anti-inflammatory compounds in our bodies. In an assessment of 1,123 people, higher levels of ALA in the blood were associated with a lower concentration of the inflammatory marker, C-reactive protein (Ferrucci *et al.* 2006). This is the mechanism by which flax seed can help relieve pain, such as arthritis.

Reduced blood platelet aggregation (that is, reduced blood clotting), and therefore improved cardiovascular disease protection, was shown in a small trial where five men consumed 40 grams of flax seed oil daily for 23 days (Allman *et al.* 1995). This appeared to be due to the omega 3 ALA in flax seed converting to another omega 3 fat called eicosapentaenoic acid (EPA) within blood platelets, which lowers blood clotting. A further six men in the trial who consumed 40 grams of sunflower seed oil, containing the omega 6 linoleic acid, did not show any improved blood clot response.

The omega 3 fat DHA, abundant in fish, is essential to a healthy brain function and is linked to reducing depression. Only a small proportion of ALA is converted to EPA and onto DHA in our bodies. However, eating the combination of flax seed, turmeric and pepper may increase the conversion of ALA to DHA (Wu *et al.* 2015).

GARLIC

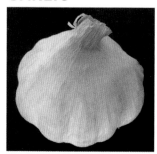 Garlic was eaten by athletes competing at the ancient Greek Olympics, establishing itself as the first performance-enhancing substance (Rivlin 2001). Garlic has been used as food and medicine for thousands of years, including by the Egyptians at least 3,500 years ago. In contrast to many other medicinally valued plants that were monopolised by the wealthy, garlic appears to have been used equally by the upper classes (being found in King Tutankhamen's tomb) and labourers, including the builders of the pyramids (Revlin 2001).

Garlic is the underground segmented bulb of the lily *Allium sativum*, which is harvested after the flowering stem dies off. It originates from central Asia and is closely related to chives, onions and leeks. Elephant garlic, *Allium ampeloprasum*, is a closely related plant with larger bulbs containing fewer segments. Recent research suggests elephant garlic is also very beneficial for our health.

Plausible health benefits
Garlic can help lower blood pressure, thin the blood, reduce blood glucose levels, lower the chance of getting a cold and relieve cold symptoms. Human studies suggest garlic has a

protective effect against cancers of the oesophagus, stomach and colon (Fleischauer & Arab 2001; Béliveau & Gingras 2014). For example, an Italian study found eating a moderate but regular amount of garlic was associated with lower chances of developing several cancers, especially of the throat (Galeone *et al.* 2006). Because garlic is a blood thinner, it is wise to consult your doctor before eating garlic or taking garlic tablets, if you are taking blood thinning or related medication. A small number of people are allergic to garlic and onions.

Significant phytochemicals

The sulphur compounds responsible for 'garlic breath' provide valuable health benefits. The inert sulphur compound alliin is present in whole garlic. Once cut or crushed, an enzyme called alliinase mixes with alliin, transforming it to the active phyto-chemical allicin. This process is very similar to the production of active sulphur compounds in cabbages, broccoli and onions following cutting. In each case, heat can destroy the enzyme responsible for producing the active compound. To allow the enzyme time to work, let garlic sit for a few minutes after crush-ing if adding to cooking. During cooking and after garlic is eaten, some allicin is further modified to other antioxidant sulphur compounds, especially diallyl disulfide.

Garlic also contains beta-carotene, the flavonoid quercetin and several lignans, for example lariciresinol. It provides vita-mins B1, B2, B3, B6, B9 (folate), C and E. Garlic has a good concentration of several important minerals including calcium, magnesium, phosphorus, potassium, selenium and zinc.

How garlic provides health benefits

Phytochemicals in garlic, especially the sulphur compound alli-cin and its derivatives, have the capacity to easily enter our cells to provide benefits (Rabinkov *et al.* 2000). A British trial found that participants taking a garlic tablet daily over winter had significantly fewer colds compared to people taking a placebo (Josling 2001). Of those in the trial who did develop a cold, people taking garlic tablets recovered faster than those who did not take garlic tablets. It is thought that the sulphur compounds and the flavonoid quercetin are primarily responsible for garlic's antiviral properties, which help protect against colds. Garlic also has valuable antibacterial and antifungal properties (Corzo-Martínez et al. 2007), and has been used as an anthelmintic in the treatment of worms.

Phytochemicals in garlic provide valuable antioxidant benefits. Quercetin in particular stimulates the production of the powerful antioxidants superoxide dismutase (SOD) and glutathione within our cells. These antioxidant properties help to prevent various diseases including some cancers, cardiovascular disease and inflammation. For example, the antioxidant properties of garlic can help reduce the damaging oxidation of the LDL 'bad' cholesterol that contributes to heart disease (Corzo-Martínez et al. 2007).

A review of 118 human studies concluded that eating garlic or taking aged garlic extracts typically provides a small but useful decrease in total cholesterol and LDL 'bad' cholesterol levels (Ackermann et al. 2001). It is thought that the sulphur compounds in garlic help to achieve this by promoting the excretion of cholesterol and reducing the amount of cholesterol made in the liver.

Sulphur compounds in garlic lead to the formation of small quantities of hydrogen sulfide, which causes the dilation of blood vessels, lowering blood pressure (Benavides et al. 2007). Garlic phytochemicals reduce the degree of clotting in the blood platelets, thereby thinning the blood (Rahman et al. 2016).

Allicin and compounds into which it converts within our bodies, such as diallyl disulfide, are known to promote the death of cells with damaged mitochondria, hence helping to prevent cancer development (Grabacka *et al.* 2014). Diallyl disulfide from garlic has been found to reduce tumour numbers in rat studies, by suppressing the protein NF-kB, which activates inflammation that can contribute to tumour development (Saud *et al.* 2016).

GINGER

Ginger is the rhizome (underground root-like stem) of *Zingiber officinale*, which has long narrow leaves growing at 90 degrees to the succulent stems. It originated in South East Asia and is a relative of turmeric and galangal. Its rhizomes can be harvested at the end of

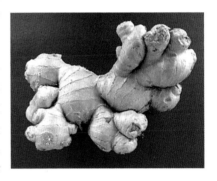

summer and also in winter when the leaves die off. The earlier, post-summer harvest provides softer rhizomes. Ginger can be eaten fresh, where it provides a sharp zing, grated to make a tea, or added as a flavouring into a huge range of recipes.

There are a few close relatives of ginger in Australia, especially native ginger (*Alpinia caerulea*), which is widely distributed in rainforests and other lush vegetation on the east coast (see Chapter 16). It has rhizomes that are reported to be edible when young (Cribb & Cribb 1990). As with other root crops, such as carrots, garlic and onions, ginger rhizomes store the plant's nutrient reserves. The rhizomes are full of healthy antioxidant and antimicrobial phytochemicals, required to protect the plant's nutrients from the multitudes of soil fungi and bacteria.

Plausible health benefits

Ginger is best known for its ability to reduce nausea, lowering the intensity of morning sickness (although it is thought best to have only one or two serves of ginger a day when pregnant) and motion sickness in many people (Thomson *et al.* 2014; Woodward 2014;

Giacosa *et al.* 2015). Ginger can be useful for improving digestion and reducing inflammation. There is evidence that ginger can help reduce the risk of developing some cancers, especially colorectal, gastric, ovarian, liver, skin, breast and prostate cancers (Mashhadi *et al.* 2013). Ginger may also be good for maintaining memory (Lim *et al.* 2014 & 2016).

Several human studies have found that ginger can provide significant pain relief. This has included relieving the pain of period cramps and osteoarthritis of the knee, sometimes as effectively as non-steroidal anti-inflammatory drugs (Altman & Marcussen 2001; Wigler *et al.* 2003; Haghighi *et al.* 2006; Ozgoli *et al.* 2009). However, one trial did not find ginger to relieve arthritic pain any better than a placebo (Bliddal *et al.* 2000).

There are suggestions that ginger promotes our immune system, making it a useful food for reducing the impacts of a cold (Schulick 2012). In Indonesia, ginger is considered useful for relieving fever (Ramdhan *et al.* 2015). It may reduce ulcers and has antifungal and antibacterial properties.

Significant phytochemicals

Ginger contains some unique and particularly beneficial polyphenols called gingerol, shogaol, paradol and zingerone (Duke 2016). When ginger is heated, some of the gingerol converts to shogaol and zingerone. It has small amounts of beta-carotene and the flavonoid quercetin (Bhagwat & Haytowitz 2015). Ginger contains vitamins B1, B2, B3, B6, B9 (folate), C and E, although in moderate concentrations. The minerals calcium, magnesium and zinc are also present.

How ginger provides health benefits

Ginger's ability to help relieve symptoms of nausea appear to be due to its affect on reducing the levels of a hormone called vasopressin (Lien *et al.* 2003). Vasopressin helps regulate water and salt in the blood and increased levels are associated with nausea. Gingerol, shogaol and zingerone also inhibit serotonin receptors in the gut, called 5-HT receptors, which appears to reduce or delay nausea symptoms (Lete & Allué 2016). Several anti-nausea drugs are based on the same action.

Phytochemicals in ginger, especially gingerol, shogaol and zingerone, have strong anti-inflammatory properties (Lakhan *et al.* 2015). They reduce inflammation, such as arthritis symptoms, by suppressing the activities of the critical inflammatory proteins, NF-kB, TNF-alpha and COX-2 (Frondoza *et al.* 2004). The half of 74 trial participants who consumed 2 grams of ginger (either raw or heated) daily for eleven days reported less pain following exercise than those taking a placebo (Black *et al.* 2010). Validating their reduced perception of pain, those taking ginger had lower levels of prostanglandin E2 in their blood, the inflammatory compound produced by the COX-2 enzyme. There is additional evidence that ginger phytochemicals (gingerols and shogaols) also reduce inflammation by inhibiting lipoxygenase (LOX) enzymes that produce leukotrienes. This is another pathway to reducing inflammation, one that is not provided by aspirin (Grzanna *et al.* 2005). Therefore, ginger supplies a multiple prong attack on inflammation.

Leukotrienes are also associated with colon cancers, suggesting another benefit of ginger's inhibition of LOX enzymes (Jeong *et al.* 2009). Laboratory research on human cells suggests gingerol and shogaol can help inhibit angiogenesis (the growth of new blood vessels) around tumours and block metastasis (the spread of cancer cells). They do this by preventing the activation of the inflammatory protein NF-kB (Hsu *et al.* 2012; Jeong *et al.* 2009).

Ginger, especially its polyphenol shogaol, has been found to help relax bronchial smooth muscle cells (Kuo *et al.* 2011). This has been shown to assist in reducing asthmatic symptoms resulting from irritation after exposure to phthalates used in soft plastic.

Ginger contributes to a healthy brain and in maintaining memory, by reducing the build-up of amyloid-beta proteins and promoting nerve growth factors (Lim *et al.* 2014; Lim *et al.* 2016).

GRAPES

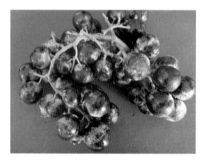

Grapes are the fruit of a vine (*Vitis vinifera*) originating from the Mediterranean region. Grapes are eaten fresh, seed oils are used, and of course grapes are fermented into wine. There are a wide number of varieties of both red and white grapes.

Plausible health benefits
Grapes are good for the cardiovascular system and may contribute to reducing the risk of developing some cancers (Lyle 2011).

Significant phytochemicals
Probably the most well-known phytochemical found in grapes is resveratrol. It is a polyphenol concentrated in grape skins, which explains why there is more in red wine (fermented with the skin) than white wines. Grapes also contain the phytosterol campesterol, and other polyphenols including ellagic and gallic acids, and a range of flavonoids such as anthocyanins, catechins (with minor amounts of epigallocatechin-3-gallate, also found in green tea), kaempferol, myricetin and quercetin (Lyle 2011). Grapes provide vitamins B1, B2, B3, B6, C and E. They contain various minerals including calcium, iron, magnesium, phosphorus, potassium, selenium and zinc.

How grapes provide health benefits
Grape phytochemicals combine to provide a strong antioxidant capacity. The cardiovascular benefits of grapes are

probably due to a combination of antioxidant and anti-inflammatory influences. Together these can reduce the oxidation damage of LDL 'bad' cholesterol, helping to reduce atherosclerosis. Grapes can also reduce blood pressure and keep blood vessels healthy, in part by stimulating nitric oxide production to relax blood vessels (Xia *et al.* 2013). Resveratrol in particular has been found to be useful in maintaining the health of blood vessels. There is also evidence that resveratrol can help inhibit tumour growth and promote cancer cell death (Xia *et al.* 2013).

GRAPEFRUIT

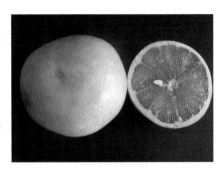

Grapefruit, *Citrus X paradisi*, are a large citrus fruit bred from hybridising an orange and a pomelo. Varieties have white, pink and red flesh (MacFarlane 2011).

Plausible health benefits

Grapefruit can help reduce excess weight and lower blood pressure. It is thought that grapefruit can also help reduce arterial stiffness, promote a stable heart rhythm and a healthy liver, and possibly reduce the development of cancers. Grapefruit affect how the liver metabolises a range of compounds, including caffeine. It is important to check with a medical doctor about possible interactions between grapefruit and medications, because grapefruit and its juice should not be consumed with some medicines.

Significant phytochemicals

All grapefruit contain the terpene limonene and red grapefruit also provide the carotenoids beta-carotene and lycopene (Craig 1997; Lyle 2011). The polyphenols present in grapefruit include bergamottin, bergapten, ferulic acid and flavonoids hesperetin, kaempferol, naringenin and quercetin. The slight bitter taste of grapefruits is due to a high concentration of naringenin (Justesen *et al.* 1998). Grapefruit supply vitamins B1, B2, B3, B9 (folate), C and E, plus fibre, magnesium and potassium.

How grapefruit provide health benefits

A study involving 77 obese people found those eating half a grapefruit three times a day before meals for 12 weeks lost more weight (1.6 kg) and showed reduced insulin resistance, compared to those not eating grapefruit, who lost 0.3 kg (Fujioka *et al.* 2006). People drinking 237 mL of grapefruit juice lost a similar amount of weight (1.5 kg) to those eating grapefruit. The study authors were unsure of the reasons for the weight loss. They speculated that because grapefruit is known to interact with liver enzymes, its phytochemicals may also interact with the production of insulin in the pancreas.

In a trial with 48 women, the half who drank 340 mL of grapefruit juice each day (providing 210 mg naringenin) for six months showed less arterial stiffness (an indicator of heart disease) than those who drank a placebo each day (Habauzit *et al.* 2015). Grapefruit have an inhibitory effect on the aggregation of blood platelets, that is they reduce blood clotting. This may reduce platelet aggregation in atherosclerotic blood vessel walls and therefore reduce the risk of heart disease (Dutta-Roy *et al.* 2001).

Grapefruit interact with cytochrome P450 enzymes in the liver, slowing the break down of various compounds. This metabolic effect can help keep a range of healthy phytochemicals in our system longer, including preventing anti-cancer compounds being eliminated too quickly (Béliveau & Gingras 2014). Eating grapefruit can also interfere with the metabolism of some medications, for example statins, leading to increased concentrations in the blood. This same mechanism may increase the uptake of caffeine or delay its degradation.

This effect is primarily due to naringenin and other polyphenol compounds called furanocoumarins, especially bergamottin (Hung *et al.* 2017). Therefore as noted earlier, it is wise to check with a medical doctor as to whether you should avoid grapefruit when taking various medications (Lyle 2011; Brunning 2015; Habauzit *et al.* 2015).

Polyphenols in grapefruit, such as bergamottin, bergapten, hesperetin and naringenin, have shown the ability to inhibit cancerous growths in laboratory trials (Hung *et al.* 2017). For example, bergapten has been found to cause the death of breast cancer cells in a laboratory (Panno *et al.* 2012).

LEMON GRASS

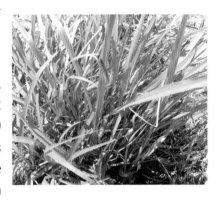

Lemon grass is a tall, tufted, citrus-scented perennial that belongs to a group of over 50 tropical grasses in the genus *Cymbopogon*. This includes nine species that grow naturally in Australia. The culinary lemon grass (*Cymbopogon citratus*) originates from the Indian region. The leaves can be used as a tea and the base of the stems of lemon grass are used in South East Asian curries.

Plausible health benefits

Externally applied lemon grass oil helps relieve itchy skin (although this must be a diluted solution so that it does not burn the skin) and is a handy insect repellent. Drinking a tea made from infused lemon grass leaves, or combining in curry, may be useful for relieving a range of health concerns including anxiety, insomnia, cold and flu symptoms and can contribute to a healthy cardiovascular system (Aggarwal & Yost 2011; Woodward 2014).

Significant phytochemicals

Lemon grass contains several flavonoids, including luteolin and quercetin. The distilled oil contains citral, limonene and 1,8 cineole.

How lemon grass provides health benefits

Citral and 1,8 cineole in lemon grass oil are antimicrobial and can repel insects. Citral has also been found to reduce inflammation by inhibiting the inflammatory-promoting enzyme COX-2 (Katsukawa *et al.* 2010). Flavonoids in lemon grass have been shown in a laboratory study to reduce the oxidative damage to LDL 'bad' cholesterol (Orrego *et al.* 2009). The combined anti-inflammatory effects and inhibition of LDL oxidation can benefit our cardiovascular system.

LETTUCE

Lettuce (*Lactuca sativa*) is a central feature in many salads. It is a type of daisy originating in Asia and is related to dandelions, echinacea and marigolds. There are a large number of cultivars of different sizes and suited to different climates.

Plausible health benefits

Lettuce contributes to a healthy diet, although there are no specific health claims for lettuce.

Significant phytochemicals

Lettuce contains beta-carotene, luteolin and quercetin (Llorach *et al.* 2008). Red lettuce has the anthocyanin, cyanidin (Rothwell *et al.* 2013). Lettuce also provides provitamin A, vitamins B1, B2, B3, B6, B9 (folate), C and E, plus calcium, magnesium and zinc.

How lettuce provides health benefits

Lettuce provides important flavonoids, vitamins and minerals, although at a relatively low level compared to many other plants. It is an important component of a healthy diet, but lettuce should be just one of many salad plants that people eat.

MACADAMIA NUTS

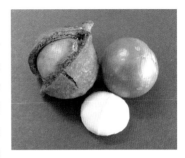

Macadamia nuts are the most abundantly grown and popular Australian bush food. The trees grow naturally in the rainforests of subtropical eastern Australia, in northern New South Wales and southern Queensland. Macadamias are part of the Proteaceae family, which includes banksias, waratahs and silky oaks. There are four different species of macadamia trees (a further three tropical Australian trees were once considered *Macadamia* species but are now in a separate genus called *Lasjia*). Only two of the four *Macadamia* species have edible nuts: *M. integrifolia* and *M. tetraphylla*. Horticultural crops of macadamia nuts are cultivars of, and hybrids between, these two species of macadamia. Sadly, the natural populations of *M. integrifolia* and *M. tetraphylla* are now considered vulnerable to extinction in the wild, primarily because of forest clearing, as well as weed invasion and inappropriate fire regimes (Costello *et al.* 2009). The Macadamia Conservation Trust works towards preserving wild populations.

Macadamia nuts are round, about 2 to 3 cm in diameter, with a thick leathery husk that splits to reveal a hard, woody brown shell. Cracking the shell to access the internal edible kernel is tricky and generations of Australians have risen to the challenge by developing a variety of tools to break through the macadamia shell. These range from hammers to cracking devices with levers. Macadamia nuts are eaten raw or roasted. Macadamia oil is a healthy and delicious cooking oil and salad dressing. Macadamias are cultivated abundantly in subtropical regions around the world, including Hawaii. Macadamia nut farms are established across eastern Australia, from the mid coast of New South Wales to the Atherton Tablelands in north Queensland.

Plausible health benefits

Macadamias are high in monounsaturated fats and eating them is considered very healthy. They can help reduce weight, lower LDL 'bad' cholesterol while maintaining HDL 'good' cholesterol levels, thin the blood and reduce inflammation, therefore helping to reduce the risk of heart disease and stroke (Lyle 2011). There is also tantalising preliminary laboratory data that they may contribute to a diet that inhibits or slows cancer development and reduces the chance of developing Alzheimer's disease. Of course, people with nut allergies must be careful with macadamias.

Significant phytochemicals

Macadamias contain several phytosterols, including campesterol and particularly good levels of beta-sitosterol (Phillips *et al.* 2005; Lyle 2011). They have a high content of healthy monounsaturated fats, especially oleic acid which is the main fat in olive oil, and palmitoleic acid. Macadamias also contain abundant soluble fibre, and vitamins B1, B3, B9 (folate), C and E. They provide a good source of magnesium, phosphorus, potassium and selenium.

How macadamias provide health benefits

The high fat and fibre content of macadamia nuts quickly relieves hunger, helping reduce over-eating. The high monounsaturated fat and phytosterol content of macadamia nuts contribute to their cardiovascular benefits. Beta-sitosterol, the most abundant phytosterol in macadamias, helps maintain a healthy cholesterol balance (Duester 2001). A variety of studies have found that regular consumption of macadamia nuts reduces total and LDL 'bad' cholesterol, while maintaining HDL 'good' cholesterol levels (Munro & Garg 2008). One trial highlighted the benefit of macadamias in lowering oxidative damage which contributes to cardiovascular disease. Seventeen men with high cholesterol ate between 40 and 90 grams of macadamia nuts daily for four weeks. Eating macadamias lowered the levels of compounds in their blood that are indicators of oxidative stress and inflammation (Garg *et al.* 2007). The men also showed reduced blood platelet aggregation - that is, macadamias helped thin their blood.

The monounsaturated omega 9 fat oleic acid, abundant in macadamias, reduces inflammation by inhibiting the protein NF-kB that triggers inflammation within our cells. Oleic acid has been found in a laboratory trial to reduce beta-amyloid peptide-induced brain nerve damage through its ability to reduce inflammation (Kim *et al.* 2015).

The phytosterol, beta-sitosterol, promotes the death of breast and prostate cancer cells in the laboratory. Phytosterols can inhibit the formation of new blood vessels around tumours (Bradford & Awad 2007).

MANGOES

The magnificent mango tree originates from India, and is named *Mangifera indica*. It is grown for its large juicy fruit in tropical and subtropical regions across the world, including Australia. Mangoes are grown in the Carnarvon region of Western

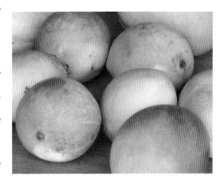

Australia, the Top End, and northern New South Wales to north Queensland (McGuire 2016). Blushing Acres, in north Queensland, have demonstrated that careful management including composting, mulching, increasing soil organic matter and fine-tuned irrigation produces particularly juicy mangoes.

Plausible health benefits

Eating mangoes can help balance blood glucose levels and contribute to the treatment or prevention of cataracts, gum disease, inflammatory pain, heart disease, macular degeneration and prostate cancer. The clear sap from mango stalks and leaves can irritate the skin and eating mangoes can cause a rash in a minor number of people.

Significant phytochemicals

Mangoes contain a smorgasbord of phytochemicals, including the carotenoids alpha- and beta-carotene, lycopene, lutein and zeaxanthin. They have a range of polyphenols including gallic acid, lupeol and mangiferin, and flavonoids proanthocyanidins, catechin, kaempferol, myricetin and quercetin. Mangoes supply provitamin A, vitamins B1, B2, B3, B9 (folate), C, E and K1, and various minerals including iron, potassium and phosphorus.

How mangoes provide health benefits

The polyphenol mangiferin, named after its original detection in mangoes, is a valuable antioxidant, with the ability to reach brain cells. Mangiferin can inhibit oxidation damage to mitochondria (which are the energy production sites within cells), therefore maintaining healthy cell function (Masibo & He 2008). The antioxidant effects of mangiferin may also be useful in the treatment of gum disease (Carvalho *et al.* 2009).

The flavonoid quercetin can reduce oxidation damage to fats, providing stability to cell membranes and potentially reducing the development of atherosclerosis. It also triggers our cells to produce the strong antioxidant glutathione. The carotenoids lutein and zeaxanthin, which contribute to the orange colour of mango flesh, are essential antioxidants that are absorbed into our eyes, where they protect against cataracts and macular degeneration.

Mangiferin provides anti-inflammatory benefits by suppressing the inflammatory protein TNF-alpha, and has been found to help stimulate the death of cancer cells in laboratory tests (Imran *et al.* 2017). Other phytochemicals present in mango flesh, especially anthocyanins, kaempferol and lupeol, can also help promote the death of cancer cells, reduce inflammation by inhibiting the protein NF-kB and relax blood vessels (Masibo & He 2008).

MULBERRIES

Mulberries are the juicy, sweet fruit of small trees with large heart-shaped leaves. There are several species of mulberry trees, which originate in Asia (white mulberry, *Morus alba*), the Middle East (black mulberry, *M. nigra*) and North America (red mulberry, *M. rubra*; McFarlane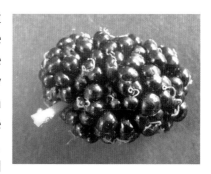
2011). The leaves of the white mulberry, and to a lesser extent black mulberry, are food for silkworms (McFarlane 2011; Lim 2012c).

Plausible health benefits

Mulberries have been used to treat inflammatory symptoms, including general pain, and contribute to cardiovascular and mental health (Lim 2012c; Liu *et al.* 2008).

Significant phytochemicals

Mulberries contain the polyphenols chlorogenic and protocatechuic acids, and flavonoids kaempferol, quercetin and taxifolin (Zhang *et al.* 2008). Black mulberries are particularly high in the anthocyanins cyanidin and pelargonidin (Powlowska *et al.* 2008).

How mulberries provide health benefits

Flavonoids in mulberries, especially the anthocyanins but also others such as taxifolin, have demonstrated strong antioxidant capacities and have been shown to reduce the oxidative damage to LDL 'bad' cholesterol in laboratory experiments (Liu *et al.* 2008; Zhang *et al.* 2008). Mulberry extracts have been shown to protect brain cells from damage by neurotoxins in a laboratory cell culture experiment and a trial using mice (Kim *et al.* 2010). The authors of this study suggested that the antioxidant capacity of mulberries was probably responsible for protecting the brain cells. They also suggested that mulberries may be able to protect nerve tissue, and that this neuroprotective affect could help treat or prevent Parkinson's disease.

OLIVES AND OLIVE OIL

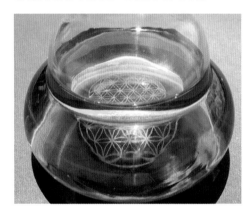

Olives (*Olea europaea*), which originate from the Mediterranean region, are one of the oldest horticultural fruit crops, dating back at least 7,000 years (Hasmi *et al.* 2015). Olive fruit are not eaten raw due to their bitter taste. The fruit are cured in salt or various liquids. Extra virgin olive oil is made by crushing the fruit and is the highest quality, while some lower grades of olive oil are produced with heat and/or chemical extraction. Olives were a staple of the ancient Greeks and olive oil remains a fundamental aspect of the healthy Mediterranean diet.

Plausible health benefits

There is good evidence that olives and olive oil reduce inflammation, lower blood pressure and reduce the risk of developing cardiovascular disease. For example, a trial involving 63 people found that consuming 20 mL of olive oil daily for six weeks led to a reduction in biomarkers that are used as indicators of cardiovascular disease (Silva *et al.* 2015). Olives and olive oil provide strong antioxidant properties and may help to reduce the chance of developing dementia, or help lower its severity. They may also reduce the risk of developing some cancers and type 2 diabetes.

Significant phytochemicals

The primary fat in olive oil is the monounsaturated, omega 9 fat oleic acid. The polyphenol oleocanthal provides the sharp taste of a good olive oil. Olives and olive oil also contain the carotenoids beta-carotene and lutein, the polyphenols hydroxytyrosol, oleuropein, p-couramic acid, resveratrol and flavonoids apigenin, diosmetin and quercetin. They supply provitamin A, vitamins B9 (folate) and E, plus minerals including calcium and magnesium.

How olives and olive oil provide health benefits

Olives and olive oil provide their health benefits through the combination of their antioxidant and anti-inflammatory effects. Several polyphenols in olive oil, including hydroxytyrosol and quercetin, are strong antioxidants. They also stimulate our cells to produce the powerful antioxidant glutathione (Rodríguez-Morató *et al.* 2015). This antioxidant capacity can reduce the free radical damage that is associated with many diseases, including dementia and cardiovascular disease. In particular, phytochemicals in olive oil help reduce oxidative damage to LDL 'bad' cholesterol, which contributes to atherosclerosis.

The sharp tasting phytochemical oleocanthal reduces inflammation and pain by inhibiting COX enzymes. This is the same process by which some pain-relieving nonsteroidal anti-inflammatory drugs work, such as ibuprofen (Beauchamp *et al.* 2005) The monounsaturated omega 9 fat, oleic acid, is also involved in reducing inflammation.

As a key component of the Mediterranean diet, regular consumption of olive oil is associated with lower rates of type 2 diabetes (Salas-Salvadó *et al*. 2010). The polyphenol oleuropein and oleic acid in olive oil each contribute to lowering blood pressure (Sun *et al*. 2017; Teres *et al*. 2008). Laboratory animal studies indicate that polyphenols and oleic acid in olive oil can promote the death of cancer cells (Fayyaz *et al*. 2016; Menendez *et al*. 2005).

Olive oil provides its full phytochemical benefit when consumed uncooked. Frying or cooking any oil at high temperatures can cause some oxidisation damage and potentially produce unhealthy compounds called aldehydes. However recent research suggests olive oil is more stable during cooking than other oils, especially compared to polyunsaturated oils, i.e. most vegetable oils (De Alzaa *et al*. 2018). This better stability during heating is provided by the high monounsaturated fat and polyphenol content of olive oil.

ONIONS

Onions (*Allium cepa*) are the bulbous base of a lily-like plant

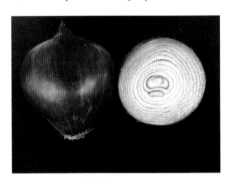

originating in Russia and the broader Asian region (McFarlane 2010). Cutting onions makes our eyes weep and sting in response to the volatile sulphur compounds that waft through the air. Rupturing onion cells allows enzymes to convert an amino acid sulfoxide into the tear-jerking sulphur compound called propanethial s-oxide (Brunning 2015). Apparently, putting an onion in the freezer briefly before cutting can slow done the reaction sufficiently to limit the tears.

Plausible health benefits

Onions are thought to enhance our immune system, with anti-inflammatory benefits that contribute to reduced allergic responses and a lower risk of cardiovascular disease (Lyle 2011). An Italian study found that eating an onion each day was associated with lower chances of developing some cancers, especially of the throat and stomach (Galeone *et al.* 2006).

Significant phytochemicals

The most characteristic phytochemicals in onions are the sulphur compounds including allicin and the tear-jerking propanethial s-oxide. Allicin can be metabolised into diallyl disulfide and diallyl trisulfide inside our bodies. The active compound allicin is produced when an enzyme within onion cells called alliinase mixes with and transforms an inert precurser to allicin, called alliin. Heat can destroy the enzyme responsible for producing the active compound. To allow the enzyme enough time to work thoroughly, it is best to let onions sit for up to ten minutes after chopping prior to cooking.

Onions also contain the phytosterols campesterol and beta-sitosterol and a range of flavonoids, especially kaempferol, myricetin and abundant quercetin (Lim 2015; Rothwell *et al.* 2013). Red onions supply the anthocyanins cyanidin and delphinidin. Onions contain vitamins B1, B2, B3, B6 and C, plus minerals including magnesium and zinc.

How onions provide health benefits

The flavonoids, especially quercetin, provide important antioxidant and anti-inflammatory benefits. They contribute to reducing blood pressure and lowering blood triglyciderides (Edwards *et al.* 2007; Egert *et al.* 2009). Quercetin can also reduce histamine levels, helping relieve hay fever symptoms. Anthocyanins, found in red onions, can enhance mental performance and help reduce the risk of cardiovascular disease and some cancers (Chen *et al.* 2006).

The sulphur compound allicin, and diallyl disulfide which it converts into within our bodies, contributes to cancer prevention. These sulphur phytochemicals can promote the death of cells with damaged mitochondria, helping to prevent cancer development (Grabacka *et al.* 2014). Diallyl disulfide has been found to reduce tumour numbers in rat studies, by suppressing the protein NF-kB, which activates inflammation that can contribute to tumour development (Saud *et al.* 2016).

PARSLEY

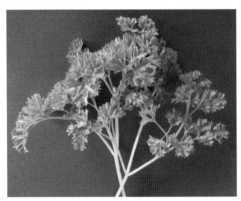

Parsley, *Petroselinum crispum*, is a herb in the carrot family (McFarlane 2010). Eating a sprig of parsley can help freshen breath.

Plausible health benefits

Parsley can contribute to cardiovascular health, lower blood sugar and possibly help relieve stomach ulcers (Aggarwal & Yost 2011).

Significant phytochemicals

Parsley contains a high concentration of the flavonoid apigenin, as well as kaempferol, myricetin and quercetin. It also has a high concentration of beta-carotene, and contains vitamins B1, B2, B3, B6, B9 (folate), C and E. Parsley supplies good amounts of calcium, iron, magnesium and potassium.

How parsley provides health benefits

The flavonoid apigenin has been demonstrated to stimulate the body to produce the antioxidants glutathione and SOD (Nielsen *et al.* 1999). It has the ability to reduce blood platelet agreggation in laboratory tests, which would contribute to cardiovascular health (Gadi *et al.* 2012).

PEAS

Peas are the seeds within the pods of a legume vine, *Pisum sativum*. They originated in the Mediterranean and western Asia, and were one of the earliest plants to be grown agriculturally. Peas are prominent in the field of genetics, because in the 1850s an Austrian monk named Gregor

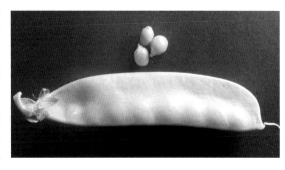

Mendel inter-bred garden peas with different characteristics to determine the process governing the inheritance of traits. His studies were fundamental in showing that each individual has two copies of what we now call genes, with a dominant and a recessive form. Unfortunately, Mendel's work went unnoticed for several decades. Mendel posted a copy of his research paper to Charles Darwin, who appears not to have opened it (Henig 2000). Mendel's work on hereditary traits would have provided Darwin with a valuable insight into a key process involved in natural selection.

Plausible health benefits

Peas may help regulate blood sugar levels, contribute to good heart health and may help inhibit the development of stomach cancer (Lyle 2011).

Significant phytochemicals

Peas contain alpha- and beta-carotenes, and the polyphenols ferulic acid, coumestrol and flavonoids apigenin, catechin, delphinidin, genistein and kaempferol (Lyle 2011; Lim 2012b). Peas also contain provitamin A, vitamins B1, B2, B3, B6, B9 (folate), C and K1. They provide good levels of protein and contain the minerals calcium, iodine, iron, nitrogen, potassium, phosphorus and zinc.

How peas provide health benefits

The antioxidant value of the phytochemicals in peas will offer benefits to the heart. The polyphenol coumestrol has been identified as a likely factor in the association between eating peas and low rates of stomach cancer (Hernández-Ramírez *et al.* 2009). Peas contain the so-called anti-nutrients lectin and phytate, as do beans, corn, flax, rice, sunflower, wheat and some other seeds (Schlemmer *et al.* 2009). Lectin and phytate can cause inflammaton and bind to some minerals, especially iron, calcium and zinc, reducing their absorption. Other components of peas (such as vitamin C) help absorb minerals, so can offset this property. Processing peas by soaking in water and cooking degrades a good proportion of lectins and phytates. These compounds do have some positive benefits, especially in binding to calcium to reduce calcification of arteries. They also provide some antioxidant capacity and perhaps anti-cancer properties (Schlemmer *et al.* 2009).

PEPPER

Pepper (*Piper nigrum*) is a small fleshy fruit with a hard seed, which is produced by a vine natural to forests of the Malabar coast of western India. It was central to the spice trade. Australia contains several native species of pepper (see Chapter 16). Black pepper is produced by harvesting the fruit before they are fully ripe and are dried with the flesh remaining, leaving a shrivelled black peppercorn. To produce white pepper, the fruit is allowed to fully ripen and the flesh removed, then dried.

Plausible health benefits

Pepper can stimulate digestion, while brief and careful inhalation of black pepper essential oil may help the process of swallowing, which is impaired in some people who have suffered a stroke (Aggarwal & Yost 2011). It is used to treat the symptoms of colds (Wangchuk 2014). Pepper may contribute to reducing the risk of developing some cancers (lung, breast and colon) and heart disease, lower the inflammation of arthritis and help reduce dementia (Aggarwal & Yost 2011). Pepper also has antimicrobial properties (Butt *et al*. 2013).

Pepper is important for increasing the bioavailability of other phytochemicals. For example, consuming pepper is critical to improving the absorption of curcumin from turmeric.

Significant phytochemicals

The alkaloid piperine provides the pungency of pepper and has been the focus of research into pepper's health properties. Pepper also contains the terpenoid oil limonene, plus polyphenols eugenol, kaempferol and quercetin (Butt *et al*. 2013; Meghwal & Goswami 2013). It supplies vitamins B1, B2, B3, B6 and E, and calcium, magnesium and potassium.

How pepper provides health benefits

Piperine can trigger our cells to make the strong antioxidant glutathione, and has been shown to cause tumour cell death in laboratory studies, that is in Petri dishes (Meghwal & Goswami 2013; Yaffe *et al*. 2015). Piperine also stimulates pancreatic enzymes, which could aid digestion. It reduces inflammation by inhibiting the production of prostaglandin E2 (Butt *et al*. 2013). Piperine interacts with liver enzymes to reduce the breakdown of curcumin, and some other phytochemicals, so that they are more available to be absorbed into the blood stream. Piperine can lower blood pressure by limiting calcium entry into blood vessel walls, preserving blood vessel flexibility (Taqvi *et al*. 2008).

POMEGRANATE

Pomegranate (*Punica granatum*) is a small tree originating from the Middle East across to India. The edible portions are the seeds and the juicy red flesh surrounding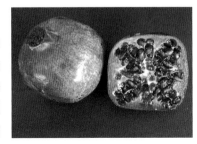

each seed. Fruit must be kept on the tree until ripe as they don't ripen after harvest (McFarlane 2011).

Plausible health benefits

Pomegranates have been used for many centuries for their medicinal properties. In particular, pomegranates can benefit cardiovascular health by helping resist the development of atherosclerosis and lower blood pressure.

Significant phytochemicals

Pomegranates contain many polyphenols including ellagic acid, the anthocyanidins cyanidin, pelargonidin and delphinidin, and other flavonoids kaempferol, luteolin and quercetin (Mertens *et al.* 2006; Bassiri-Jahromi 2018). They contain vitamins B1, B2, B3, B6, B9 (folate), C and E, plus calcium, magnesium and potassium.

How pomegranates provide health benefits

Within half an hour of drinking a pomegranate extract, there are detectable levels of ellagic acid and enhanced antioxidant capacity in the blood (Mertens *et al.* 2006). Drinking pomegranate juice has repeatedly been found to have cardiovascular health benefits. One study found benefits in drinking 240 mL of pomegranate juice daily for up to 18 months in participants with the most severe signs of cardiovascular disease. These findings did not apply to those with less severe symptoms, however (Davidson *et al.* 2009). Specifically, drinking pomegranate juice slowed the progression of carotid intima media thickness. This is a way of assessing the inner two layers of the carotid artery, and thicker measurements are an indicator of atherosclerosis (the build-up of plaque), and the risk of heart disease and stroke.

Another amazing but small trial found that pomegranate juice is capable of reopening narrowed carotid arteries by around a third. Ten people with severe carotid artery stenosis (a narrowing of the carotid arteries in the neck by 70 to 90%, typically due to atherosclerosis) drank 50 mL of pomegranate juice (diluted 1:5

with water) daily for one year. They showed ongoing improvements over the twelve months, and after one year the narrowing of their neck arteries had reduced by an average of 35% (Aviram *et al.* 2004). They also had reduced blood pressure, and their LDL 'bad' cholesterol had less damage from oxidation. Another nine patients who drank a placebo rather than pomegranate juice developed a further 9% increase in blockage of their carotid arteries by the end of the year (Aviram *et al.* 2004). The authors suggested that the antioxidant properties of the polyphenols, including anthocyanins, contained in the pomegranate juice were responsible for the observed benefits.

In a further trial, involving 45 people with heart disease, half of the patients drank pomegranate juice for three months. These patients showed improved blood flow, with less symptoms of ischaemia (reduce blood flow to the heart) during exercise or other stress tests. Ischaemia increased over the three months in the other half of the patients, who were not drinking pomegranate juice (Sumner *et al.* 2005).

QUINOA

Quinoa (*Chenopodium quinoa*) is the seed of a plant in the Chenopodiaceae family, which includes beetroots, spinach and the Australian saltbushes. Quinoa originates in low rainfall, high altitude areas of South America, such as Bolivia. It is cooked in water and used in similar ways to rice, as well as made into a flour.

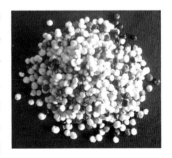

Plausible health benefits

While not a true grain (which are seeds of grasses, such as corn and rice) quinoa is generally considered a very healthy seed, or pseudograin. Being unrelated to wheat, quinoa does not contain gluten and therefore quinoa flour is a good substitute for people who are gluten intolerant. Quinoa can contribute to eye and cardiovascular health, promote healing, reduce oxidation damage to cells and help limit inflammation, including inflammatory pain (Noratto *et al.* 2015).

Significant phytochemicals

Quinoa seeds provide carotenoids beta-carotene, lutein and zeaxanthin, and polyphenols ferulic acid and flavonoids kaempferol and quercetin (Tang & Tsao 2017). They contain phytoecdysteroids, which are phytochemicals that are chemically similar to insect hormones that promote moulting (shedding of exoskeletons in insects). Quinoa is a good source of various amino acids, used as the building blocks for proteins. It contains vitamins B1, B2, B3, B6, B9 (folate) and E. Quinoa is a good source of calcium, iron, magnesium, selenium and zinc. The seed coat of quinoa contains phytate and saponins. Both phytate and saponins can have health values if consumed at low levels, such as binding to overabundant metals that can cause oxidative damage to our eyes (Adams 2014). However, saponins and phytate can reduce nutrient absorption and potentially cause stomach pain. Quinoa seeds must be soaked (with the water then discarded) prior to cooking, which removes a good proportion of phytate and perhaps a little of the saponins (Lyle 2011).

How quinoa provides health benefits

Beta-carotene, lutein and zeaxanthin are important antioxidants, especially contributing to healthy eyes. The polyphenols in quinoa, such as flavonoids, reduce inflammation by inhibiting the activation of the inflammation-triggering protein NF-kB (Noratto *et al.* 2015). Phytoecdysteroids have been found to promote growth and healing of broken bones, improve glucose metabolism and reduce the development of atherosclerosis in mice (Lafont & Dinan 2003).

RASPBERRIES, BLACKBERRIES, BRAMBLES AND LOGANBERRIES

Raspberries and their relatives black-berries, boysenberries, loganberries and youngberries, are various species and cultivars of prickly vines and scrambling bushes within the genus *Rubus*. Raspberries are *Rubus idaeus*, blackberries *R. fruticosus* and *R. ulmi-folius*, while boysenberry, loganberry 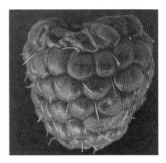 and youngberry are considered hybrid cultivars from various species of *Rubus* (McFarlane 2011). Australia has several native species of *Rubus*, such as *R. moluccanus* (see Chapter 16). Several northern hemisphere *Rubus* species and cultivars have become aggressive land degrading weeds in Australia, especially blackberries, so that care is needed to limit their unwanted spread when cultivating them. They are successful as invaders because they are able to produce new plants from segments of stems that touch the ground, and they germinate abundantly from seeds that are widely dispersed by birds.

Plausible health benefits

Raspberries and blackberries may help reduce blood glucose levels and provide relief from cold symptoms (Patel *et al*. 2004; Wangchuk 2014). Their phytochemicals likely provide strong antioxidant and anti-inflammatory benefits, potentially reducing the risk of developing cardiovascular disease and some cancers.

Significant phytochemicals

Raspberries and their cousins provide a range of flavonoids, including anthocyanins (cyanidin, delphinidin and pelargoni-din), catechins, kaempferol, myricetin and quercetin (Patel *et al*. 2004; Rothwell *et al*. 2013). They also contain ellagic, gallic and p-coumaric acids and vitamins B1, B2, B3, B6, B9 (folate) and C. Raspberries provide the minerals calcium, magnesium and selenium.

How raspberries provide health benefits

The broad range and high concentration of phytochemicals in raspberries provide strong antioxidant and anti-inflammatory benefits. Laboratory experiments of cultured cells have found that raspberry extracts can reduce oxidation of fats and inhibit the inflammatory-causing enzyme COX-2. They can also hinder the growth of cultured tumour cells (Bowen-Forbes *et al.* 2010).

Raspberries can slow the absorption of glucose from food into the blood by reducing the production of a digestive enzyme called alpha-amylase (McDougall *et al.* 2005). Slowing the rate of glucose absorption into the blood is important in limiting glucose over-supply and reducing insulin spikes.

RICE

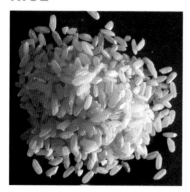

Rice is the seed of the grass *Oryza sativa*, which originates from South East Asia. Australia hosts several native species of wild rice. Cultivated rice grows naturally in wetlands and hence is typically planted in rice paddies, where flooded conditions can be maintained. The establishment of broad-scale rice cultivation provided a substantial quantity of food that helped enable the development of large communities and civilisations throughout Asia. This was the equivalent to the cultivation of wheat in the Middle East and corn in South America.

Plausible health benefits

Rice is a significant source of starch and hence energy. Brown rice contributes to cardiovascular health. It does not contain gluten, so can be a staple grain for coeliacs and people who have some intolerance of wheat. However, rice does contain other gluten-like lectins that may be a problem to some people.

Significant phytochemicals

Whole, unrefined brown rice contains many polyphenols such as caffeic, ferulic and p-coumaric acids, and flavonoids including anthocyanins, luteolin and tricin. Brown rice also contains the omega 6 fat linoleic acid and omega 9 fat oleic acid (also in olives), vitamins B1, B2, B3, B6, B9 (folate) and E, and good amounts of magnesium, zinc and fibre. Many of the nutrients are present in the outer husk of rice, which is retained in brown rice. Refined white rice has a considerable proportion of the nutrients removed in processing. This has led to the development of the disease beriberi in some people eating only white rice (which lacks vitamin B1).

How rice provides health benefits

Many phytochemicals in rice, especially ferulic acid and anthocyanins, provide antioxidant properties. The fibre in rice helps promote healthy gut microbes. Brown rice increases the proportion of HDL 'good' cholesterol in the blood, while reducing LDL 'bad' cholesterol and triglycerides levels. These effects, combined with the antioxidants in rice, contribute to improved cardiovascular health (Lyle 2011).

Brown rice has a lower glycaemic index than white rice, meaning that glucose levels in the blood rise more slowly, reducing insulin spikes.

ROSEMARY

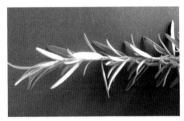

Rosemary (*Rosmarinus officinalis*) is a woody herb from the Mediterranean, able to be propagated into new plants from stem cuttings (McFarlane 2010). Its leaves add flavour to a range of dishes and act as a food preservative. The oils from rosemary leaves are used in aromatherapy.

Plausible health benefits

The essential oils (diluted) from rosemary are used externally on the skin as an antiseptic and for relaxing muscles (Lyle 2011). Eating rosemary leaves may reduce hay fever allergy symptoms and may also improve blood flow by relaxing blood vessels.

Significant phytochemicals

Rosemary contains several terpene oils, including beta-pinene, camphor, carnosol, cineol and limonene. It also contains beta-carotene, the polyphenols ferulic and rosmarinic acid (also found in mint and sage) and flavonoids apigenin, hispidulin and naringenin. Rosemary provides provitamin A, vitamins B1, B2, B3, B6, B9 (folate) and C, plus calcium, magnesium and zinc.

How rosemary provides health benefits

The phytochemical carnosol, also found in sage, is a strong antioxidant. Rodent studies indicate that carnosol can reduce the oxidatve damage to LDL 'bad' cholesterol and activate the powerful antioxidant, glutathione (Johnson 2011). Due to the strong antioxidant properties of rosemary phytochemicals, especially carnosol and rosmarinic acid, seasoning meat with rosemary leaves dramatically reduces the production of potentially carcinogenic heterocyclical amines that form during high temperature cooking of meat (Puangsombat *et al.* 2011).

A clinical trial involving 21 people found a reduction in the allergy symptoms of itchy eyes and nose in the subgroup of patients taking rosmarinic acid extract (Osakabe *et al.* 2004). The researchers felt that the extract reduced the allergy symptoms because it can lower the number of polymorphonuclear leukocytes (a white blood cell) accumulating in the nostrils, and inhibits the inflammatory enzyme COX-2.

Consuming a rosemary extract for 21 days improved blood vessel function, with better blood flow, in 19 volunteers of a study in Slovenia (Sinkovic *et al.* 2011). The researchers felt it likely that the improved blood vessel function resulted from the antioxidants in rosemary, especially carnosol and rosmarinic acid.

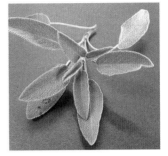

SAGE

Sage (*Salvia officinalis*) and the closely related Spanish sage (*Salvia lavandulaefolia*) are herbs of the mint family with greyish, wrinkly leaves. They have a long European history of use as a herb and tea.

Plausible health benefits

Sage is especially known for its effect on improving memory, alertness and mood, as well as helping digestion and to relieve sore throats (Shipard 2003; Aggarwal 2010). Both sage and Spanish sage have been shown to enhance memory and mood and reduce anxiety in human trials (Tildesley *et al.* 2005; Kennedy *et al.* 2006; Scholey *et al.* 2008). Sage may also reduce excessive sweating (Castleman 2017). It probably also provides similar benefits to its close relative rosemary – that is, it may help reduce hay fever symptoms and improve blood flow.

Significant phytochemicals

Sage contains the polyphenols carnosol and caffeic, rosmarinic and vanillic acids, and flavonoids apigenin, luteolin and quercetin, all of which are powerful antioxidants. The herb also contains the carotenoids beta-carotene and lutein. Sage contains some of the highest concentrations of many of the B vitamins found in plants (B1, B2, B3, B6, B9), as well as supplying vitamins C and E and provitamin A. It offers good concentrations of the minerals calcium, iron, magnesium and zinc, as well as the omega 3 fat alpha-linolenic acid (ALA).

How sage provides health benefits

Researchers believe that sage improves memory and mood through a combination of mechanisms. In one interaction, the neurotransmitter acetylcholine, which promotes attention, is degraded more slowly. Sage does this by inhibiting the enzyme acetylcholinesterase, which breaks down acetylcholine (Tildesley *et al.* 2005; Kennedy *et al.* 2006). Several of the phytochemicals in sage, especially rosmarinic acid (also in rosemary) provide protection to brain cells by reducing oxidation damage and promoting brain derived neurotrophic factor (Iuvone *et al.* 2006; Lopresti 2017).

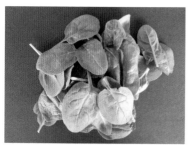

SPINACH

Spinach is an annual herb (*Spinacia oleracea*) originating in the Middle east (MacFarlane 2010). The leaves are eaten raw or steamed. Spinach is related to beetroot and quinoa (all in Chenopodiaceae).

Plausible health benefits

Spinach is highly regarded as a healthy vegetable. It may contribute to boosting mental performance, reducing blood pressure and lowering the risk of developing dementia, cataracts and macular degeneration.

Significant phytochemicals

Spinach leaves contain the carotenoids lutein and zeaxanthin, the phytosterol coumestrol and the flavonoids kaempferol and myricetin (Sultana & Anwar 2008). Young 'baby spinach' leaves have been found to have a higher concentration of some flavonoids than older leaves (Bergquist *et al.* 2005). Spinach contains provitamin A, vitamins B1, B2, B3, B6, B9 (folate), C and E, plus minerals such as magnesium and potassium.

How spinach provides health benefits

Spinach leaves are a good source of lutein and zeaxanthin, which are important antioxidants for protecting the eyes, reducing the chance of developing cataracts and macular degeneration. A trial with 108 people suffering early stages of macular degeneration found that supplementation with 20 mg of lutein, or 10 mg each of lutein and zeaxanthin daily for 48 weeks improved macular pigment and indicators of vision (Ma *et al.* 2012). A cup of cooked spinach provides 20 mg combined total of lutein and zeaxanthin (Linus Pauling Institute - http://lpi.oregonstate.edu/book/export/html/52 accessed 11 February 2018). Lutein and zeaxanthin may also boost brain performance. A trial that provided 51 young adults with 10 mg of lutein and 2 mg of zeaxanthin supplements daily demonstrated that spatial memory was improved after a year (Renzi-Hammond *et al.* 2017).

Spinach provides plenty of nitrates, and human studies indicate that the nitrates can be converted to nitric oxide, which reduces blood pressure (Gee & Ahluwalia 2016). Spinach leaves have a reasonably high concentration of oxalic acid (oxalates). Oxalates can bind to some minerals, reducing their absorption. This includes calcium, and kidney stones are made of calcium oxalate. People with kidney problems, or who are susceptible to kidney stones and potentially even muscle cramps, should be careful not to eat too much spinach. Steaming or boiling leaves can reduce oxalates to an extent.

STRAWBERRIES

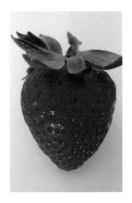

Strawberries are the fruit of a spreading ground cover plant (*Fragaria × ananassa*), which is in the same family as roses (the similarities can be seen in the strawberry's white flowers, which resemble older rose varieties). They are a hybrid, developed in France, from two species of *Fragaria* and plants are propagated by runners (i.e. stem shoots) to ensure that the fruit remain consistent. The tiny pips on the outside of the fruit are the seeds. Strawberries are grown from south Western Australia through south eastern Australia to north Queensland, with about a third of Australia's crop grown on the Sunshine Coast (McGuire 2016).

Plausible health benefits

There is evidence that long-term consumption of strawberries slows the development of cognitive decline in older people. Strawberries can help lower blood glucose levels, benefit cardio-vascular health, and may contribute to inhibiting the development of some cancers. Strawberries have antimicrobial effects that may help to keep teeth and gums healthy (Lyle 2011; Devore *et al.* 2012).

Significant phytochemicals

Strawberries provide a smorgasbord of phytochemicals. These include the polyphenols ellagic, chlorogenic and p-coumaric acids, and flavonoids including anthocyanins (cyanidin, pelargonidin and procyanidin), catechin, kaempferol, myricetin and quercetin. Strawberries also contain vitamins B1, B2, B9 (folate), C, and the minerals magnesium, phosphorus and potassium.

How strawberries provide health benefits

A trial involving 23 healthy men and women found that eating 500 grams of strawberries daily for a month reduced LDL 'bad' cholesterol by 13.7% and lowered triglycerides in the blood by 20.8%, while maintaining the level of HDL 'good' cholesterol. This trial also showed strawberries thinned the blood by reducing blood platelet clustering (Alvarez-Suarez *et al.* 2014). After a month of strawberry feasting, the participants had increased plasma antioxidant capacity. The researchers attributed these effects to the high levels of vitamin C and flavonoids, especially anthocyanins, in the strawberries.

Drinking a strawberry drink containing the equivalent of 110 grams of strawberries has been found to reduce the oxidation damage to LDL 'bad' cholesterol after people ate a high fat meal (Burton-Freeman *et al.* 2010). In another study, 16 women with metabolic syndrome drank two cups of strawberry juice daily for a month, confirming strawberries reduce the levels of, and oxidative damage to, LDL 'bad' cholesterol (Basu *et al.* 2009). Reductions in markers of inflammation in the blood, C-reactive protein and interleukin-6, have been documented within hours of eating strawberries (Edirisinghe *et al.* 2011).

The digestive enzyme alpha-amylase is found in saliva and in the small intestines. It breaks down starches, such as in bread, into glucose units to be absorbed into the blood. Strawberries can slow the absorption of glucose from food into the blood by reducing the amount of alpha-amylase produced (McDougall *et al.* 2005). By slowing the rate of glucose absorption, the process reduces the pressure on the insulin response to limit glucose over-supply within the blood.

Information collected from the long-term Nurses' Health Study suggests that older people who eat blueberries and strawberries display a slower decline in cognitive performance (Devore *et al.* 2012). The anthocyanins in strawberries probably contribute to this benefit, through their antioxidant and anti-inflammatory properties.

Ellagic acid, found in strawberries, helps detoxify carcinogens by enhancing phase 2 detoxification enzyme activities in our liver. It has also been found in laboratory studies to activate a protein called p53, which promotes the death of cancer cells (Sakulnarmrat 2012; Riaz *et al.* 2017).

TEA

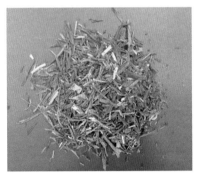 Broadly speaking, tea is a drink made by the infusion of plants in hot water. Tea can be made from a wide range of plants, including peppermint and lemon myrtle. However, the word tea usually refers to the drink made by infusing processed young leaves of the shrub *Camellia sinensis* (related to the *Camellia* flowers grown in gardens), which originated in China.

The cultivation and distribution of tea has a colourful past. For example in 1848 the Englishman Robert Fortune travelled through China, disguised as a local, to steal seeds and the secrets of tea processing on behalf of the British East India Company (Rose 2010). This horticultural espionage removed China's monopoly on tea, spurring the cultivation of tea plants across the tropics, especially in India and Sri Lanka.

Black, green and oolong tea come from the leaves of the same tea plant. Green tea is made by steaming freshly harvested leaves and then immediately drying them, usually by heating, to prevent oxidation. The preparation of black tea involves turning moist leaves over for an hour or two to allow some oxidation (often called tea fermentation) before heating and drying. This oxidation turns the leaves a dark colour and alters the chemistry of some polyphenols. Oolong tea is in between green and black tea, and is given a small amount of oxidation time before drying.

Plausible health benefits

Habitual tea drinking improves cardiovascular health, through its antioxidant protection of blood vessels, and by reducing blood pressure and improving blood flow through blood vessel dilation. Tea enhances mental function and may help treat or reduce the risk of developing type 2 diabetes (Binosha *et al.* 2017). Tea, especially green tea, may help people to manage and reduce weight. Drinking tea may contribute to the prevention of several cancers, such as breast and prostate cancers (Grabacka *et al.* 2014).

Significant phytochemicals

Both green and black teas contain the alkaloids caffeine and theophylline. Tea is a major source of polyphenols for many people, providing gallic acid and a range of flavonoids, such as anthocyanins, quercetin and especially catechins, including epigallocatechin-3-gallate. Black tea is higher in caffeine, gallic acid and theaflavins than green tea (Jochmann *et al.* 2008). Theaflavins are the products of catechins altered during the oxidation process used to produce black tea. Green tea has a higher concentration of catechins, including epigallocate-chin-3-gallate. Tea also contains small amounts of vitamin B9 (folate) and iodine.

How tea provides health benefits

Tea plants make health-boosting flavonoids to protect them-selves from oxidative damage and as a defence against disease. For example, the antimicrobial properties of their flavonoids, especially catechins, protect tea plants from diseases such as fungal blister blight of their leaves (Punyasiri *et al.* 2004). These antimicrobial properties of flavonoids in tea help protect our stomach and intestines from disease-causing microbes.

Human trials indicate that various catechins are rapidly absorbed into our blood, including the most studied and probably the most beneficial, epigallocatechin-3-gallate. The antioxidant capacity of human blood plasma increases significantly within half to one hour of drinking a cup of black or green tea (Serafini et al. 1996). There is some evidence that drinking tea without milk provides a greater antioxidant potential, possibly due to the interaction of polyphenols with milk proteins, but this effect may be minimal (Serafini et al. 1996).

One of the alkaloids in tea, theophylline, is used in some asthma bronchodilator medications. Trace amounts of theophylline are also created when the liver metabolises caffeine. Theophylline opens the airways in the lungs to make it easier to breathe (Sharangi 2009).

Drinking tea, especially green tea, may help with weight management, probably by lowering appetite and reducing glucose absorption from the gut, while increasing energy expenditure and fat burning (Rains et al. 2011). For example, a study involving 35 people with metabolic syndrome found that the participants drinking four cups of green tea a day over eight weeks reduced their weight by an average of 2.5 kg more than those drinking hot water (Basu et al. 2010). A separate study found improved weight loss by combining the consumption of catechins in tea with exercise (Maki et al. 2009).

The polyphenols in tea increase the antioxidant capacity in our blood and cells by activating the transcription protein Nrf2. This stimulates our cells to make the powerful antioxidants glutathione and superoxide dismutase, SOD (Frei & Higdon 2003). At the same time, the polyphenols in tea reduce inflammation by inhibiting the actions of the gene transcribing protein NF-kB, which triggers the production of inflammatory compounds. In this way, tea can contribute to relieving inflammatory problems such as irritable bowel syndrome (Farzaei *et al*. 2015).

A Japanese study following 40,000 adults over 11 years found that people who regularly drank green tea had a lower incidence of cardiovascular disease (Kuriyama *et al*. 2006). Drinking tea helps improve cardiovascular health in several ways. The antioxidants help reduce oxidative damage to LDL 'bad' cholesterol and blood vessels. Drinking green tea has been found to encourage a healthy ratio of HDL 'good' cholesterol to LDL 'bad' cholesterol (Basu *et al*. 2010). Tea also improves blood flow. For example, within two hours of drinking either black or green tea, blood vessel dilation increased considerably in a study of twenty-one women. This appeared to be caused by the tea polyphenols (especially catechins and theaflavins) stimulating nitric oxide to relax blood vessel muscles (Jochmann *et al*. 2008). Associated with this, long-term tea drinking (both black and green teas) reduces blood pressure (Liu *et al*. 2014).

Drinking tea, especially green tea, is associated with a lower risk of developing several cancers, including of the breast, colon and prostate (Wilkinson 2015). A Japanese study of 472 women with breast cancer found that women with phase 1 and 2 breast cancer had fewer axillary lymph node metastases when drinking green tea. Unfortunately, this effect did not apply to women with phase 3 cancer (Nakachi *et al*. 1998). Of particular interest, epigallocatechin-3-gallate in green tea has been found to promote the death of cancer cells in laboratory studies (Azam *et al*. 2004; Grabacka *et al*. 2014).

Tea probably enhances mental function by improving blood flow, and by supplying caffeine. Tea polyphenols possibly slow the formation of beta-amyloid plaques that contribute to Alzheimer's disease (Binosha *et al*. 2017).

TOMATOES

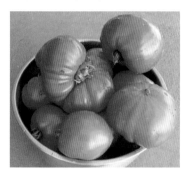

Tomatoes are a significant crop grown and appreciated across the world. Tomatoes are the fruit of *Lycopersicon esculentum*, which originated in South America. They are part of the nightshade (Solanaceae) family, which includes chillies, eggplants and potatoes. Depending on the cultivar, tomato plants may grow as a bush or a vine (McFarlane 2010). Organically grown tomatoes have been found to contain higher concentrations of the health-promoting flavonoids kaempferol and quercetin than tomatoes grown with pesticides and artificial fertilisers (Mitchell *et al.* 2007). This is probably because plants make phytochemicals in response to insect attack and phytochemicals can be promoted with good levels of soil organic matter, but reduced by high levels of nitrogen fertilisers.

Many of the compounds that provide tomatoes with their flavour are associated with important nutrients (Goff & Klee 2006). Some modern cultivars appear to have lower concentrations of flavour compounds than older varieties (Tieman *et al.* 2017). Tomatoes also lose some of their flavour when stored in the fridge because several of the flavour compounds are destroyed by storing at 4° C (McGuire 2016; Zhang *et al.* 2016).

Plausible health benefits
Tomatoes may contribute to reducing the risk of developing breast, lung and prostate cancers (Béliveau & Gingras 2014; Wilkinson 2015). They may also help reduce the risk of heart disease (Dutta-Roy *et al.* 2001).

Significant phytochemicals
Tomatoes contain a wealth of useful phytochemicals, including a range of carotenoids, especially beta-carotene, lycopene, lutein,

phytoene and zeaxanthin (Lyle 2011). Lycopene provides their red colour. They also contain many flavonoids such as kaempferol, naringenin and quercetin, as well as other polyphenols, caffeic acid, chlorogenic acid, p-coumaric acid and resveratrol (Slimestad & Verheul 2009).

Tomatoes provide provitamin A, vitamins B3, B9 (folate), C and E, and the minerals calcium, magnesium, phosphorus, potassium and zinc. They contain the protein lectin, which can bind to minerals to reduce their absorption, and can potentially promote inflammation in some people who may be better off avoiding tomatoes. Cooking tomatoes can degrade a proportion of their lectins and can increase the availability of the health-promoting carotenoids.

How tomatoes provide health benefits

Tomato extracts have been found to have anti-inflammatory properties, through the inhibition of the protein TNF-alpha (Navarrete *et al.* 2015). Tomatoes (especially the juicy part of the fruit) are an effective inhibitor of blood platelet aggregation (i.e. clotting), potentially reducing the risk of heart disease (Dutta-Roy *et al.* 2001). Several trials have found significantly reduced platelet aggregation in blood collected after people drank tomato extract (Dutta-Roy *et al.* 2001; O'Kennedy *et al.* 2006).

Tomatoes may also reduce the oxidation of prostate tissue and therefore could provide a valuable contribution to the treatment of prostate cancer (Flores-Perez & Rodriguez-Concepcion 2012). The lycopene in tomatoes is anti-angiogenic, meaning it inhibits the development of new blood vessels around tumours (Wilkinson 2015). Tomato juice has been shown to reduce indicators of oxidation, with the lycopene content reducing total cholesterol (Jacob *et al.* 2008). As lycopene is a fat-soluble compound, it is best absorbed when mixed with fats, such as olive oil. As mentioned earlier, cooking makes carotenoids, such as lycopene, more bioavailable.

It does this by breaking plant cell membranes to release lycopene from inside the cell compartments.

TURMERIC

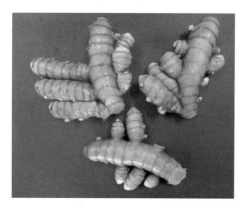

Turmeric (*Curcuma longa*) is the orange rhizome (i.e. root) of a ginger-like plant that grows naturally throughout tropical Asia. There is a close relative (*Curcuma australasica*) on Cape York Peninsula in northern Australia that is said to be edible after roasting (Cribb & Cribb 1990). Turmeric rhizomes store the plant's nutrient reserves when the leaves die off over the dry season (winter). It is the rhizomes that are used to propagate new plants. These are full of healthy antioxidant and antimicrobial phytochemicals, which protect the plant's nutrients from the multitudes of soil fungi and bacteria.

Turmeric is a key ingredient in curries and can be grated raw onto salads or cooked in a huge range of vegetarian and meat dishes. To get the full benefit of turmeric, it is best to eat it with fats such as olive oil, and pepper which dramatically increases the absorption of curcumin (a key active compound in turmeric) into our blood.

Plausible health benefits

Turmeric has been used medicinally for thousands of years, especially in Indian Ayurvedic medicine, and has many health benefits attributed to it. For example, people who regularly eat turmeric tend to have relatively low rates of several cancers, especially of the breast, colon and prostate (Sinha *et al.* 2003; Goggins & Wong 2009; Ali *et al.* 2010). Eating turmeric may help in the treatment of allergies, anxiety, arthritis, asthma, cholesterol imbalance, depression, type 2 diabetes, gout and stomach ulcers. It is reported to help with weight management, and in reducing the risk of developing heart, liver and Parkinson's diseases, as well as assisting recovery after stroke (Lyle 2011; Aggarwal & Yost 2011; Fanaei *et al.* 2016). A crushed piece of turmeric can be applied to cut skin to help in wound healing and it can help soothe psoriasis (Woodward 2014). Applying turmeric powder directly to swollen gums or rinsing the mouth with turmeric powder mixed with cloves in water, may be useful for healing gums and reducing dental pain (Sambhav *et al.* 2014). Note that because turmeric can help thin the blood, medical advice should be sort about whether to consume it with some medications.

Significant phytochemicals

The spicy smell of turmeric is provided by aromatic compounds called turmerones. Turmeric also contains alpha-santalene (found in allspice), beta-carotene, zingiberene (also found in ginger) and curcumin. Curcumin is a polyphenol that provides the orange colour of turmeric and has received the most research attention (Yadav *et al.* 2013; Flores 2017). Turmeric contains other curcumin-related compounds such as cyclocurcumin and demethoxycurcumin. A high proportion of curcumin is modified in the liver into curcumin sulphate and curcumin glucuronide, with some being split into smaller compounds such as ferulic acid and vanillin (Toden & Goel 2017). These altered versions of curcumin also provide health benefits. Eating turmeric with pepper greatly enhances the proportion of curcumin that is absorbed unmodified into the blood stream, due to the influence of pepper's phytochemical, piperine, limiting the liver's tendency to modify curcumin (Shoba *et al.* 1998).

Turmeric also contains provitamin A, vitamins B1, B2, B3, B6, B9 (folate), C and E. It has high concentrations of various minerals including iron, magnesium, selenium and zinc.

How turmeric provides health benefits

Phytochemicals in turmeric, such as curcumin and turmerones, have antioxidant properties which extinguish free radicals that cause cell damage. This antioxidant function is especially effective through the digestive tract, helping our throats, stomach and intestines. They are also stimulators of the protein Nrf2, which promotes the production of the powerful antioxidants glutathione and superoxide dismutase (SOD) within our cells. Combined, these antioxidant actions lower the chance of developing various diseases such as Alzheimer's, and reduce the oxidative damage to LDL 'bad' cholesterol that contributes to atherosclerosis and therefore to heart disease and stroke.

The anti-inflammatory properties of turmeric can reduce painful conditions such as arthritis. In a trial involving 120 people, turmeric extract was shown to reduce the pain of arthritis of the knee (Madhu *et al.* 2013). Another trial involving 367 people found that turmeric extract provided a relief from arthritic knee pain to the same degree as that provided by the common pain-relieving drug ibuprofen (Kuptniratsaikul *et al.* 2014). Curcumin reduced pain and fatigue in patients recovering after laparoscopic cholecystectomy surgery - removal of the gall bladder through a small incision (Agarwal *et al.* 2011). Curcumin and other curcuminoids in turmeric reduce inflammation by suppressing the protein NF-kB, thereby reducing production of the inflammatory compound prostaglandin E2 (Sharma *et al.* 2004; Sandur *et al.* 2007).

Turmeric is receiving considerable research attention for its potential to contribute to the prevention of some cancers, such as of the breast, colon and prostate. Laboratory trials of turmeric and curcumin extracts demonstrate that it can inhibit the formation of new blood vessels around tumour cells, and promote tumour cell death (Kim *et al.* 2014). These anticancer functions are complemented by the ability of turmeric phytochemicals to reduce inflammation (Park *et al.* 2012; Wilkinson 2015).

A recent study has found one mechanism by which turmeric promotes the death of cancer cells. Laboratory research established that curcumin selectively inhibits a protein in our cells called DYRK2 (Banerjee *et al.* 2018). As a result, it impedes the actions of another protein called proteasome 26s, which is involved in removing damaged proteins from cells. By blocking DYRK2, and therefore inhibiting proteasome 26s, curcumin causes the accumulation of damaged proteins within cancer cells, which can lead to their death (Béliveau 2018). The inhibition of proteasomes is the mode of action provided by some cancer drugs.

One human trial investigated the role of curcumin in the recovery of patients following colon cancer surgery. Of the 126 participating patients, 106 received post-operative radiotherapy and/or chemotherapy. Half of the 126 patients took 360 mg curcumin capsules three times daily prior to and after surgery, for a total of 10 to 30 days. Patients taking curcumin regained more weight, and their blood showed greater reductions in the inflammatory protein TNF-alpha and higher levels of the protein p53. This protein promotes the death of diseased cells, and there were more dead tumour cells in the colon tissue of patients taking curcumin (He *et al.* 2011).

It has been found that curcumin-free extracts of turmeric suppress tumour growth in mice, indicating that several phytochemicals in turmeric, in addition to curcumin, contribute to its potential cancer preventative benefits (Prasad *et al.* 2017). The aromatic oils in turmeric, the turmerones, provide antioxidant and anti-inflammatory health benefits and improve curcumin absorption, indicating the benefits of eating whole (or powdered) turmeric rather than, or in addition to, taking curcumin extracts (Verma & Kuma 2017). Seasoning meat with turmeric reduces the production of potentially carcinogenic heterocyclical amines that form during high temperature cooking (Puangsombat *et al.* 2011).

Further research is needed to determine the extent to which turmeric can inhibit cancer development and progression in people, before conclusions can be made (Gibson-Moore & Spiro 2017). Laboratory trials, such as those described above, have determined mechanisms by which turmeric and curcumin extracts can inhibit cancer cells cultured in Petrei dishes. This demonstrates turmeric has the potential to contribute to cancer prevention. While caution is needed not exaggerate the current limited knowledge about turmeric, it warrants further assessment into how it can contribute to cancer treatment (Gupta *et al.* 2013).

Turmeric can provide powerful benefits to our digestive system, because our throat, stomach and intestines are exposed to turmeric phytochemicals before any are metabolised in the liver. For example, a trial involving 45 patients with stomach pains found that eating 3 grams of turmeric powder (in capsules) daily for twelve weeks healed the ulcers in 19 of the 25 patients who had ulcers of the stomach or small intestine. The remaining 20 patients in the trial lacking a detectable ulcer also experienced relief from stomach pain after four weeks of taking turmeric (Prucksunand *et al.* 2001). The authors felt turmeric's anti-inflammatory actions, by inhibiting the protein NF-kB, were responsible for healing the ulcers and general stomach pain. Its anti-inflammatory benefits are thought to be of great potential for helping patients with inflammatory bowel disease (Ali *et al.* 2012).

Turmeric may provide some assistance in reducing the symptoms of type 2 diabetes because it can help reduce the oxidative and inflammatory damage to blood vessels that a constant high blood glucose can cause (Flores 2017).

Phytochemicals in turmeric contribute to improved cardio-vascular health in several ways. They reduce the oxidative damage to LDL 'bad' cholesterol, which can lead to athero-sclerosis, and turmeric thins the blood by reducing blood platelet clumping (Labban 2014). Reduced blood platelet aggregation is achieved by inhibiting the production of throm-boxane, which is the same mechanism by which aspirin thins the blood. Turmeric can reduce the absorption of fats from a meal by inhibiting the actions of fat digesting enzymes (McCrea *et al.* 2015). Curcumin has been found to lower uric acid levels in the blood of patients with non-alcoholic fatty liver disease (Panahi *et al.* 2016). It may therefore help relieve gout symptoms.

In rat studies, consumption of curcumin is linked to improved nerve cell size within the hippocampus area of the brain. Curcumin may promote a protein called brain-derived neurotrophic factor (BDNF), which is important in the growth and survival of brain cells (Flores 2017). A recent study using rats as subjects found that curcumin increased the conversion of the omega 3 fat from flax seed, ALA, to the DHA omega 3 used in their brains (Wu *et al.* 2015). Deficiencies in DHA are linked to anxiety and dementia.

A study involving people over the age of 60 with pre-diabetes found improved working memory (that is, better recall in tests) in 23 participants who ate turmeric. In comparison, 22 participants not taking turmeric showed no memory improvement (Lee *et al.* 2014). The authors suggested that the memory improvements may be due to turmeric's ability to reduce inflammation, or improve communication between nerves and perhaps mitochon-drial function.

The aromatic turmerones have anti-microbial and antifungal properties, which probably contribute to wound healing benefits and may help reduce microbe infections in the gut.

WATERCRESS

Watercress (*Nasturtium officinale*) is a peppery-tasting herb of wet areas, with small, slightly glossy rounded leaves. It is a plant of the cabbage family, originating in Europe and Asia (MacFarlane 2010). Watercress can become a weed of some wetlands due to its abundant seed germination capacity, so care is needed to contain the spread of plants.

Plausible health benefits

It is likely that watercress contributes to a diet that reduces the chance of developing some cancers, cataracts and macular degeneration.

Significant phytochemicals

Watercress is a good source of the carotenoids beta-carotene, lutein and zeaxanthin and the sulphur compounds phenethyl isothiocyanate (PEITC) and indole-3-carbinol (I3C; Lyle 2011; Pandey *et al.* 2018). Heat damages the enzyme myrosinase that catalyses the activation of PEITC and I3C, so that watercress should only be cooked briefly, if at all. Watercress provides provitamin A, vitamins B1, B2, B3, B6, B9 (folate), C and E, plus minerals including calcium, iodine, iron, magnesium and zinc.

How watercress provides health benefits

The carotenoids in watercress, especially lutein, provide important antioxidant benefits to our eyes, reducing the chance of developing cataracts and macular degeneration. The sulphur compounds PEITC and I3C have been found in numerous laboratory trials to inhibit the proliferation of tumours (Navarro *et al.* 2011). These two compounds achieve this through several mechanisms, including enhancing the removal of carinogenic toxins, inhibiting the inflammatory-promoting protein NF-kB and promoting the death of tumour cells.

WATERMELON

Watermelons are a quintessen-
tial summer fruit. They are the
football-sized fruit of the vine
Citrullus lanatus var. *lanatus.*
Originating in Africa, watermelons were grown thousands of
years ago by Egyptian and Chinese people.

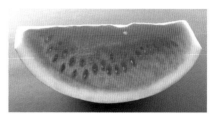

Plausible health benefits

Watermelons help reduce muscle soreness after exercise and
may help reduce the risk of developing some cancers.

Significant phytochemicals

The red colour of watermelon flesh is mainly due to the abundance of
lycopene, which is the same phytochemical that makes tomatoes red.
Watermelon contains other carotenoids, alpha- and beta-carotenes
and lutein, and the polyphenols caffeic acid and flavonoid luteolin.
Watermelons contain provitamin A, vitamins B1, B2, B3, B6, C and
the amino acid citrulline. They provide a variety of minerals including
calcium, iodine, iron, magnesium, phosphors potassium and zinc.

How watermelons provide health benefits

A trial with eleven men found that watermelon juice improved
heart rate recovery after exercise and reduced muscle soreness,
apparently via the amino acid citrulline (Tarazona-Díaz *et al.*
2013). The anti-inflammatory effects of phytochemicals will
contribute to this benefit. The carotenoid lycopene, mostly studied in tomatoes, shows potential for reducing the risk of developing some cancers, especially prostate cancer. This effect of
lycopene is especially due its capacity to limit new blood vessel
growth around tumours.

Chapter 16
Phytochemicals in Australian native bush food plants

Australia, New Zealand and New Guinea have ancient biological links with India, South America and Africa, from when they were joined together as part of the Gondwanan landmass millions of years ago. A more recent biogeographic link to South East Asia has developed with the Australian continental shelf's current proximity to Indonesia. As a result of this shared past, Australia is home to many plants that are closely related to those that have made an important contribution to history. These include relatives of all the main spices: pepper, nutmeg, cinnamon, cloves, turmeric and ginger, as well as bananas, citrus and rice.

A few Australian plants are close relatives of significant pharmaceutically active plants such as cocaine bush (*Erythroxylum* species). Many have demonstrated valuable pharmaceutical benefits. This includes corkwood (*Duboisia myoporoides*), which although toxic is a source of the alkaloid drugs scopolamine and hyoscyamine purified for dilating pupils for eye surgery, and hyoscine is employed as a medication for seas sickness (Cribb & Cribb 1988; Collins *et al.* 2004). Recently, a compound (tigilanol tiglate) extracted and purified from the poisonous fruit of blushwood (*Fontainea picrosperma*) by northern Australian researchers at QBiotics, has proved to be valuable in treating external tumours in animals (Boyle *et al.* 2014). The compound is currently under human trials.

Aboriginal and Torres Strait Islander peoples of Australia thrived on the plant and animal foods across the Australian continent and islands for thousands of years. Regular burning practices were used in many locations to maintain a healthy landscape that provided game and plant foods. A myriad of plants were eaten, many requiring detailed knowledge of how to neutralise or remove toxins. This traditional knowledge of which plants are edible and how to prepare them is an expertise for which Aboriginal and Torres Strait Islander peoples deserve respect and acknowledgement.

The health benefits of Australian native food, including meat, was highlighted in a significant study in the early 1980s. Nutritional researcher Kerin O'Dea documented the health benefits of a return to traditional life and food by ten Aboriginal people from Derby, in north Western Australia. The ten people, all of whom suffered from diabetes, left urban life and returned to a hunting and gathering lifestyle on their traditional lands for seven weeks. Professor O'Dea documented an average weight loss of 8 kg, and greatly improved blood glucose, insulin and triglycerides levels in all ten people by the end of the seven weeks. Their improved insulin levels were attributed to weight loss, a low-fat diet (64% of energy was obtained from low fat wild meat) and increased physical activity (O'Dea 1984).

Early European explorers and botanists documented plant foods used by Aboriginal people and trialled many plant foods themselves. In particular, the explorer Ludwig Leichhardt was a regular taste-tester of plants he came across and was a detailed note taker. Early European settlers also used plants that reminded them of plants from Europe, including the apparent use of the fruit of some hopbushes (*Dodonaea* shrubs) in brewing, because they (vaguely) resemble hops.

Some excellent research by CSIRO and Australian university scientists over recent decades has delved into the medicinal properties of Australian plants. Researchers from Griffith (in collaboration with Queensland Herbarium botanists), New South Wales, Queensland, South Australia and Southern Cross Universities have been particularly active in this field (e.g. Cock & Mohanty 2011; Konczak *et al.* 2012; Semple *et al.* 1998; Wohlmuth *et al.* 2007). Research into Australian plants for medicines has also been undertaken by smaller organisations, including the anti-tumour potential of tigilanol tiglate from blushwood, mentioned earlier. The distilled oil from tea trees (*Melaleuca alternifolia*) is well respected for its antiseptic qualities. However, there is much less known about the health benefits of Australian bush foods compared with conventional fruits, vegetables, herbs and spices.

The Australian native food industry is growing in quantity and quality. The most commonly cultivated Australian food plants, beside macadamia nuts, include Davidsonia plums (*Davidsonia* species), finger limes (*Citrus australasica*), lemon myrtle (*Backhousia citriodora*), native bush pepper (*Tasmannia lanceolata*) and the red quandong (*Santalum accuminatum*). Research into their phytochemicals and potential health benefits is an expanding field. Studies have focused on a few key plants, such as Davidsonia and Kakadu plums, especially by Izabela Konczak and her team at the Universities of New South Wales and Queensland. Vic Cherikoff's (2015) 'Wild Foods' book highlights the value of this and other research, indicating that several Australian plant foods have exceptional phytochemical properties.

Kakadu plums (*Terminalia ferdinandiana*), reported to be useful for relieving headaches and cold symptoms, contain very high levels of vitamin C and beneficial polyphenols such as ellagic acid (Chaliha *et al.* 2017). Davidsonia plums (three species of *Davidsonia*) have high anthocyanin levels (Konczak *et al.* 2012). Australian flora include important plants that have only been subjected to limited research and should be considered valuable food, spice and medicinal plants of the future. Breeding programs using Australian native wild rices may improve the heat tolerance of cultivated rice (Henry *et al.* 2010).

There are hundreds of edible Australian plants (although many of these are toxic until prepared appropriately). This chapter provides a summary of recent research into the phytochemical properties and potential health benefits of a subset of Australian bush foods. The information focuses on the species for which there is available phytochemical information, or are close relatives of other plants across the world with known phytochemical content. It provides suggestions on their likely health benefits, based on the known effects of the phytochemicals they contain. For readers looking for information on a broader range of Australian edible plants, there are many excellent books and websites (for example see https://anfab.org.au).

Australian native plants, and their produce, should be sourced from reputable horticultural growers and produce suppliers. These include north Queensland suppliers Rainforest Bounty near Malanda and Rainforest Heart near Millaa Millaa, Green Harvest in southern Queensland, Daley's fruit tree nursery in New South Wales and Diemen Pepper in Tasmania (see for example https://anfab.org.au for a larger list of suppliers). It is not recommended that you eat fruit, leaves or tubers etc. from plants in the wild. Absolute caution would be required before tasting any plants growing in the wild because the required certainty in identification can be difficult; many plants that look similar to bush foods are highly poisonous. The correct identification is essential and even then, some varieties of an edible species may be toxic. Also, many plants are toxic if not prepared properly (such as by cooking or lengthy soaking in water). Indeed, caution is needed when trying any new food, because some people are allergic to many commonly eaten plants.

This chapter takes the approach that the known health benefits of specific phytochemicals, determined through research on other plants, will likely provide similar benefits where present in Australian bush foods. This is of course the approach taken when nutritionalists describe the health benefits of vitamins and minerals present within various fruit and vegetables. That is, the benefits of vitamin C are generally considered the same, whether it comes from citrus, capsicums or Kakadu plums. However, it is clear many phytochemicals work synergistically and until further research is undertaken, we cannot be sure how other components of Australian bush foods will interact with the effects of various phytochemicals. Therefore, the information presented about the potential health benefits of plants in this chapter is speculative, with less confidence than can be provided for many conventional fruit and vegetables that have been the subject of more thorough research.

Key Australian edible bush food plants and their phytochemicals

Anise myrtle (*Syzygium anisatum* - previously named *Backhousia anisata*) is a tree of rainforests in northern New South Wales. It is closely related to lemon myrtle and the lilly pillies. Their leaves have a wavy edge and new leaves have an attractive red colouration. The trees are cultivated for their leaves, which are used as a tea, as a source of aniseed flavouring and for their distilled oils (RIRDC 2014a).

No specific health benefits are known to have been recorded historically for anise myrtle. However, the phytochemicals in anise myrtle probably provide valuable antioxidant and anti-inflammatory roles. Anise myrtle provides vitamins B9 (folate), C and E, the polyphenols chlorogenic and ellagic acids and flavonoids myricetin and quercetin (Konczak *et al.* 2012; Konczak 2015). It also contains calcium, iron, magnesium and zinc.

In a laboratory study, anise myrtle leaf extract inhibited the activity of an enzyme called alpha-glucosidase, which helps promote the absorption of glucose in our gut (Konczak *et al.* 2012). This means anise myrtle leaves could potentially slow glucose absorption and help lower blood glucose levels.

The presence of the strong antioxidant and anti-inflammatory quercetin in anise myrtle suggests it could help reduce inflammation, including arthritis. It may also inhibit excessive production of histamine, which is involved with allergic reactions, and help thin the blood. Myricetin is known (from research into other plants) to help reduce blood pressure and prevent atherosclerosis by limiting oxidation of LDL 'bad' cholesterol (Salvamani *et al.* 2014). Studies using mice as research subjects suggest that myricetin promotes mitochondria in their work to produce energy in muscle cells, thereby improving physical endurance (Jung *et al.* 2017). Ellagic acid, also found in several cultivated berries, has been shown to help reduce blood vessel growth around tumours and help to detoxify carcinogens by enhancing some phase 2 detoxification enzyme activities (Labrecque *et al.* 2005; Sakulnarmrat 2012). Anise myrtle extracts have been found to reduce the proliferation of cancer cells cultured in a laboratory study (Sakulnarmrat *et al.* 2013).

Bakul (*Mimusops elengi*) is a coastal tree of northern Australia and the Pacific Islands. It also grows naturally in India, where the fruit and concoctions made from the bark are considered to have medicinal properties. Eating the flesh of the bakul fruit may provide useful antioxidant benefits and is thought to help relieve diarrhoea and headaches (Roqaiya *et al.* 2015). Bakul fruit contain ellagic acid and other polyphenols, plus the phytosterol beta-sitosterol, which is also abundant in avocados (Boonyuen *et al.* 2009).

Extracts of bakul fruit show antioxidant capabilities in the laboratory (Boonyuen *et al.* 2009). Ellagic acid is known for its antioxidant properties. Beta-sitosterol reduces the absorption of cholesterol (Duester 2001) and promotes the death of breast and prostate cancer cells in laboratory tests (Bradford & Awad 2007).

Beach almond (*Terminalia catappa*) is a tree of beach dunes, growing naturally in northern Australia and many tropical areas, including India. It is a relative of Kakadu plum (*Terminalia ferdinandiana*). The inner seeds contain phytosterols and the flavonoids kaempferol and quercetin, which provide antioxidant properties (Cock 2015). Note that the fruit of some other *Terminalia* species are toxic.

Bulkuru (*Eleocharis dulcis*), also called Chinese water chestnut,

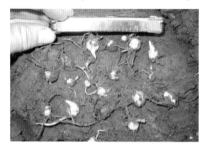

is a sedge with bulbs that are edible after roasting. It grows in wetlands across northern Australia and through South East Asia. Bulkuru supplies several health-promoting flavonoids, including apigenin (common in parlsey), fisetin, galangin (also found in galangal), luteolin and quercetin (Zhan *et al*. 2016). Bulkuru flavonoids are good antioxidants, which can promote the death of lung cancer cells cultured in laboratory experiments (Zhan *et al*. 2016). Quercetin can help reduce inflammation, potentially helping to lower the pain of arthritis (Lakhanpal & Rai 2007).

Burdekin plum (*Pleiogynium timorense*) is an attractive tree of

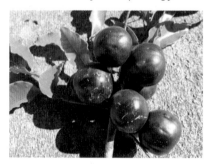

drier types of rainforest and lush watercourses in north eastern Australia, New Guinea, Timor and a few Pacific islands. The fruits have a thin outer fleshy layer over a hole-dotted hard seed coat. Burdekin plums have a fairly high anthocyanin content (especially cyanidin 3-glucoside) which contributes to the purple colour of the skin (Netzel *et al.* 2007). Anthocyanins evaluated in more commonly grown fruit, such as berries, provide antioxidant and anti-inflammatory benefits, which can enhance mental performance and help reduce the risk of cardiovascular diseases and some cancers (Chen *et al.* 2006).

Bush tomatoes are the fruit of several native species of Solanum, especially *Solanum centrale, S. chippendalei* and *S. ellipticum* (Vincent 2010). Note the fruit of many other Solanums are toxic. *Solanum centrale* contains the polyphenols chlorogenic, ferulic and hydroxybenzoic acids and kaempferol and quercetin (Konczak *et al.* 2009). These phytochemicals provide valuable health benefits. For example, chlorogenic acid contributes to reducing the oxidation of LDL 'bad cholesterol' and quercetin is a strong antioxidant and an inhibitor of inflammation with anti-histamine properties.

Conkerberries, currant bushes (*Carissa laxiflora, C. lanceolata, C. ovata and C. scabra*) are widespread spiny shrubs, the latter three with juicy edible black fruit (Cribb & Cribb 1988), which can cause diarrhoea if eaten in excess and are poisonous if not completely ripe. Broken stems and unripe fruit exude a white sap containing cardiac glycosides, toxins 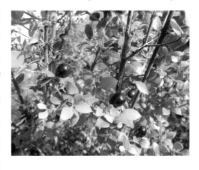 that act on the heart (McKenzie 2012). *Carissa laxiflora* grows in beach forests and it is not known whether its fruit are edible. *C. ovata* (also called *C. spinarum*) grows in eucalypt forests and rainforests along the east coast, *C. lanceolata* is common across inland northern Australia and *C. scabra* is a rainforest shrub. Their African relative, *C. edulis*, is used to treat many ailments including headaches and toothaches, and shows antioxidant and anti-viral properties (Al-Youssef & Hassan 2017; Fowsiya & Madhumitha 2017). It is possible that the fruit of Australian species of *Carissa* have similar antioxidant benefits, though no research has been undertaken on them yet.

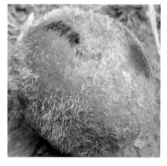

Davidsonia plums (*Davidsonia jerseyana, D. johnsonii* and *D. pruriens*) are rainforest trees that grow naturally on the east coast of Australia. Wild populations of *Davidsonia jerseyana* are only known from rainforest in northern New South Wales. *Davidsonia johnsonii* grows in rainforests straddling northern New South Wales and southern Queensland. Both *Davidsonia jerseyana* and *D. johnsonii* are rare in the wild. *Davidsonia pruriens* originates from the rainforests of north Queensland. All three species are cultivated, although *D. pruriens* is the most commonly grown commercially. Davidsonia plums are dark blue and about 4 to 6 cm in diameter. The edible flesh of the fruit is quite tart and is therefore not typically eaten raw. In addition, *D. pruriens* has irritating hairs on the surface of the fruit that must be removed before eating. Davidsonia plums are cooked and made into popular jam and savoury condiments. There is a single, old report of a person vomiting and having epigastric pain after eating unripe, raw Davidsonia plums (Flecker 1945, referred to in Hegarty *et al.* 2001). Uncooked plums contain cyanogenic glycosides that release hydrogen cyanide when chewed, and possibly other unidentified toxins (McKenzie 2012). Cyanogenic glycosides are also present in some commonly eaten fruit such as passionfruit.

Davidsonia plums (*Davidsonia pruriens*) contain phytochemicals with antioxidant and anti-inflammatory potentials greater than blueberries (Sakulnarmrat 2012). *Davidsonia pruriens* contain the carotenoid lutein, the flavonoids myricetin, quercetin and several anthocyanins in high concentrations, especially cyanidin-3-sambubioside and delphinidin (Netzel *et al.* 2007;

Konczak *et al.* 2012). Similar anthocyanins in blueberries are thought to enhance the growth and survival of brain neurones and to have an important role in learning and memory. In one laboratory trial, a fruit extract of *D. pruriens* inhibited the proliferation of cancer cells in a Petri dish almost as well as blueberry extract (Sakulnarmrat *et al.* 2015). In another laboratory study, *D. pruriens* extract was found to inhibit the activity of alpha-glucosidase, an enzyme that helps promote the absorption of glucose from our food (Konczak *et al.* 2012). This means that *D. pruriens* fruit can potentially slow glucose absorption and help keep blood glucose levels low.

Lutein is essential for eye health and has been shown to help mental performance, for example increasing the processing speed of visual information (Bovier & Hammond 2015). The flavonoids myricetin and quercetin provide important antioxidant and anti-inflammatory benefits. Combined, the phytochemicals present in Davidsonia plums likely make it a healthy fruit of particular value to our mental capacities (although these benefits may be offset if large amounts of sugar are mixed with Davidsonia plums during jam production).

Figs are shrubs and trees, some of which begin life as an epiphyte growing on other trees, eventually strangling the host. They produce soft round fruits that develop with the pollinating aid of a wasp. Several Australian species of *Ficus* are edible, including *Ficus coronata*, *F. opposita*, *F. platypoda* and *F. racemosa*. The cultivated fig (*F. carica*), originating in the Mediterranean and western Asian regions, contains the flavonoids anthocyanin and quercetin, and the terpene lupeol (Lyle 2011; Voung *et al.* 2014). Various studies have shown that these phytochemicals provide antioxidant and anti-inflammatory properties and can help to inhibit the development of cancer cells. Australian figs may also provide these benefits.

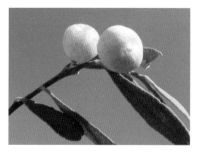

Finger limes and other Australian native citrus (*Citrus australasica, C. australis, C. garrawayi, C. glauca, C. gracilis* and *C. inodora*). *Citrus glauca* (pictured) and *C. gracilis* are spiny bushes growing in woodlands, with *C. glauca* growing mostly inland from the east coast and across to South Australia, and *C. gracilis* growing in the Top End of the Northern Territory. *Citrus gracilis* has a Near Threatened status due to its limited numbers in the wild. The other native *Citrus* species grow naturally in rainforests of the east coast of Australia. *Citrus inodora* from the wet tropics has a small distribution and is considered vulnerable to extinction in the wild.

Finger limes (*C. australasica*) are the most commonly cultivated Australian native citrus. They have been found to contain citric acid, limonene (in the peel), the carotenoid lutein, vitamins B9 (folate), C and E and decent amounts of the minerals calcium, magnesium and potassium (Konczak 2015). The red variety of finger limes also contains the anthocyanins cyanidin 3-glucoside and peonidin 3-glucoside (Netzel *et al.* 2007). An analysis of *C. inodora* fruit juice found it to contain the flavonoid naringin-6"-malonate (Berhow *et al.* 1998).

The flavonoids in native citrus will likely provide considerable antioxidant and anti-inflammatory health benefits. Flavonoids in oranges and other commonly cultivated citrus contain many flavonoids that probably also occur in Australian native citrus, such as hesperetin. This flavonoid has been shown to help limit inflammation by inhibiting the over-expression of the protein COX-2, and to help lower allergic reactions by reducing the release of histamine (Tsujiyama *et al.* 2013). The anthocyanins detected in red fruited finger limes may contribute to healthy brain function by reducing oxidation and inflammation.

Limonene, which provides the characteristic citrus smell, helps stimulate the detoxification process. The carotenoid lutein, present in finger limes, provides essential antioxidant protection to our eyes, reducing the risk of developing cataracts and macular degeneration.

Gotu kola (*Centella asiatica*) is a herb related to parsley that grows in moist areas. It has round heart-shaped leaves about the size of a 20 cent piece, with slightly toothed margins. It spreads horizontally by sending 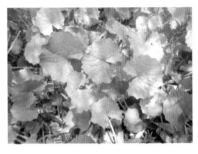 out roots at nodes along the stems. Gotu kola grows naturally in most states of Australia, and throughout Asia, many Pacific Islands and Africa. It can easily be mis-identified and confused with other plants, so it is best to source plants from a reputable supplier.

Gotu kola leaves have been used as a traditional medicine in many countries, especially China and India (Ayurvedic medicine), to boost memory and brain function, relieve anxiety and arthritis, and to improve circulation (Williams 2013; Woodward 2014). One or two leaves are usually chewed or made into a tea. Fresh or dried leaves can be applied externally to help heal wounds and soothe skin rashes (Cribb & Cribb 1988; Woodward 2014). Although side effects are rare, it is thought prudent to only consume a leaf or two a day and that pregnant women and young children should not ingest gotu kola (Castleman 2017). Gotu kola can cause photosensitivity in some people (Woodward 2014). Like many physiologically valuable plants, gotu kola may interfere with medications, such as blood thinners including warfarin, warranting medical advice before using (Williams 2013).

Gotu kola contains fat-soluble terpenes called centellosides (including asiaticoside and madecassoside), beta-carotene, various polyphenols including the flavonoids apigenin, kaempferol, myricetin and quercetin, and vitamin C (Bevege 2004; Orhan 2012). Experiments show that fertilising with nitrogen, phosphorus and potassium increases gotu kola leaf size but reduces the concentration of asiaticosides (Müller *et al.* 2013).

The leaves of gotu kola have high antioxidant capacities, due to their polyphenol content (Zainol *et al.* 2003). These antioxidant benefits appear to contribute to the reported improvements in mental performance. Water extracts of gotu kola increase antioxidant responses in mice brains, associated with improved spatial memory (Gray *et al.* 2016). Researchers have found direct human evidence of brain-boosting benefits in several trials using extracts of gotu kola. Mental performance and mood were improved in healthy elderly people, and also elderly people with mild cognitive impairment (Wattanathorn *et al.* 2008; Tiwari *et al.* 2008). Extracts of gotu kola inhibit an enzyme responsible for the break-down of the neurotransmitter acetylcholine, which is the mechanism targeted by some Alzheimer's drugs (Orhan 2012). Acetylcholine plays an important role in learning, memory and motor function, therefore slowing its degradation can be useful for our cognitive health.

Asiaticoside and flavonoids, such as quercetin, in gotu kola may help reduce allergic reactions by inhibiting histamine release and reducing the actions of the inflammatory-promoting protein NF-kB (Jiang *et al.* 2017). Some people have observed that chewing a few leaves of gotu kola daily can relieve arthritis pain. This is most likely the result of asiaticoside and the flavonoids kaempferol and quercetin inhibiting NF-kB.

The wound healing benefits of gotu kola typically occur from the application of leaves or extracts externally to wounds, but eating a small number of gotu kola leaves or their extracts, can also help (Bylka *et al.* 2014). One trial examined the benefits of consuming asiaticoside extracted from gotu kola (50 mg of asiaticoside per capsule) on wound healing in diabetic adults. Eighty-four diabetic patients took two capsules of gotu kola extract three times per day with meals, while 86 patients took placebo capsules, without any gotu kola extract. Those taking the gotu kola extract demonstrated more rapid wound healing and reduced scarring (Paocharoen 2010). The author felt this was due to gotu kola enhancing collagen production and reducing inflammation.

Grasses The seeds of several Australian grasses were an important source of food to many Aboriginal people, being edible after processing by such means as grinding and baking (Pascoe 2014). These include native millets (*Echinochloa turneriana* and *Panicum decompositum*), kangaroo grass (*Themeda triandra*), sorghums (e.g. *Sarga leiocladum*) and wild rices (*Oryza australiensis*, *O. meridionalis* and *O. rufipogon*). Some of these native Australian grasses have been found to have considerable nutritional values. For example, Australian wild rices have higher levels of several minerals, such as nitrogen, calcium, magnesium and zinc than cultivated brown rice, *Oryza sativa* (Wurm *et al.* 2012). Cultivated rice contains several beneficial phytochemicals, such as anthocyanins and luteolin. It is likely that wild rice contains many of the same phytochemicals with their associated health benefits.

The leaves and stems of Australian lemon grasses (especially *Cymbopogon ambiguus* and *C. obtectus*) and lemon grasses from other countries have been used as teas to relieve symptoms of chest infections, headaches, muscle cramps and sore eyes (Avoseh *et al.* 2015; Cribb & Cribb 1988; Grice *et al.* 2011). The commonly cultivated lemon grass (*C. citratus*), which originates from South East Asia, contains the polyphenols caffeic and chlorogenic acids and flavonoids apigenin, kaempferol and quercetin (Avoseh *et al.* 2015). The Australian lemon grass *C. ambiguus* contains the terpenoid oils eugenol and elemicin, which have been found to inhibit factors associated with headaches. They can reduce blood platelet aggregation and promote the release of serotonin 5-HT (Grice *et al.* 2011). The researchers found that eugenol inhibited the inflammatory-causing COX-2 enzyme to the same level as aspirin. Eugenol is also present in nutmeg and cloves, and is useful for relieving toothaches. Eugenol and elemicin are probably also present in several other *Cymbopogon* species.

Several native grasses have the potential to provide valuable, healthy food crops, with the benefit that many are perennial species that maintain top-soil structure (Pascoe 2014). From an ecological perspective, Australian grasses contribute much of the plant diversity in many eucalypt forests and woodlands, and of course grasslands. However, the abundance of numerous Australian native grasses has declined considerably over the last century. Australian native grasses can be conserved in their ecosystems through a number of actions, depending on the location and threat. These include reducing the smothering impact from introduced exotic pasture grasses, implementing regular, low intensity burning under mild conditions with good soil moisture, and keeping the combined grazing pressure from livestock and native herbivores to a moderate level.

Herbert River cherry (*Antidesma bunius*) is a small rainforest tree with separate male and female plants, and broad, alternatively arranged leaves with minute translucent dots (Cooper & Cooper 2004). It grows in scrub and lush creeks in north Queensland, from the Herbert River near Ingham north to Weipa. It also grows naturally in New Guinea and across South East Asia. The edible fruit (yellow to red) of Herbert River cherry have long fruit stalks, similar to normal cherries, although they are not related. The fruit were once the subject of an experiment into differences in taste perception published in the prestigious journal Nature. Apparently 39% of the 170 taste-testers found a Herbert River cherry extract slightly sour, 23% sweet, 17% salty, 15% found it bitter and the others could not describe the taste (Henkin & Gillis 1977).

The Herbert River cherry is considered of medicinal importance in Thailand, where it is called Mao Luang and is thought to be helpful in treating stomach upsets and diabetes (Butkhup & Samappito 2008). The cherries contain several flavonoids, anthocyanins, catechins (also abundant in tea), myricetin, procyanidin B1 and B2 (also found in peaches and plums) and quercetin (Butkhup & Samappito 2008; 2011; Jorjong *et al.* 2015). Other polyphenols, caffeic, ellagic and gallic acids, are also found in the cherries (Butkhup & Samappito 2011). These phytochemicals in Herbert River cherry provide a strong antioxidant capacity (Butkhup & Samappito 2011).

Illawarra plums, also known as brown pine, (*Podocarpus elatus*) are the fruit of an Australian native pine tree that grows in rainforest and other lush vegetation along the east coast from New South Wales to north Queensland. The fleshy purple, edible 'fruit' are actually enlarged stalks to each seed. The related, shrubby dwarf pine plum (*P. spinulosus*; pictured) also has edible fruit (Cribb & Cribb 1988; Darren 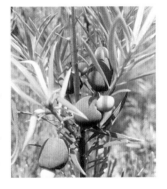 Burns pers. com. 2016; Caton & Hardwick 2016). Illawarra plums are high in anthocyanins, especially cyanidin but also delphinidin and pelargonidin, with quercetin also present (Tan *et al.* 2011a). Extracts of Illawarra plums inhibit the production of the inflammatory prostaglandin E2 in laboratory experiments (Tan *et al.* 2011b). Another laboratory experiment found that Illawarra plum extracts reduce the proliferation of colon cancer cells in Petri dishes (Symonds *et al.* 2013). The abundance of anthocyanins in Illawarra plums are likely to provide similar health benefits as those in blueberries and cherries, including stimulating our cells to create the strong antioxidant glutathione. They may also contribute the brain boosting effects that anthocyanins in other fruit provide.

Kakadu plums (*Terminalia ferdinandiana*) are fruit from a small tree that grows in tropical eucalypt woodlands in northern Australia, from the Kimberley across to Cape York Peninsula. Its fruit are a traditional food of Aboriginal people of the region (Brock 1997), who mainly eat the flesh of the fruit. The seeds are also said to be edible but contain some toxins, so it is best not to eat the seeds at all, or limit the number eaten (RIRDC 2014b).

The antioxidant and anti-inflammatory benefits of Kakadu plums are likely to provide a wide range of health benefits. These may include contributing to prevention of, or delaying, Alzheimer's disease, cardiovascular disease, cancer and type 2 diabetes (RIRDC 2014b).

Wild growing Kakadu plums have one of the highest recorded levels of vitamin C, which is crucial for a range of functions in our bodies, including the creation of collagen and as a strong antioxidant (Netzel *et al.* 2007). They also supply vitamins B9 (folate) and E, the carotenoid lutein, and polyphenols gallic and ellagic acids and flavonoids hesperetin, kaempferol, luteolin and quercetin (Mohanty & Cock 2012; Konczak 2015). Kakadu plums contain a range of minerals including calcium, iron, magnesium and zinc (Konczak 2015).

The combination of fat-soluble antioxidants (e.g. lutein and vitamin E) plus water soluble antioxidants (e.g. vitamin C and flavonoids) in Kakadu plums provide broad antioxidant bene-fits (Konczak 2015). The high levels of vitamin C and E, plus other phytochemicals in Kakadu plums give them a stronger antioxidant potential than blueberries (Konczak *et al.* 2010). Laboratory experiments of Kakadu plum extracts on cultured cells indicate that some of its antioxidant benefits are due to the activation of the protein Nrf2, which is known to stimulate our cells to produce the strong antioxidant glutathione (Tan *et al.* 2011b).

Kakadu plum phytochemicals have anti-inflammatory effects by inhibiting the enzyme COX-2, thus limiting the production of prostaglandin E2 (Tan *et al.* 2011b). This is the same mechanism by which aspirin reduces inflammatory pain.

The carotenoid in Kakadu plums, lutein, is known to protect our eyes from oxidative damage, reducing the chance of developing cataracts and macular degeneration. The flavonoids hesperetin and quercetin can help reduce allergic reactions by inhibiting the release of histamine. Kakadu plums also show antibacterial benefits (Cock & Mohanty 2011).

Lemon aspen is the fleshy, aromatic fruit of the tree *Acronychia acidula*, which originates in rainforests of north Queensland and is now cultivated in orchards. Similar to its citrus relatives, its leaves have small translucent oil dots that provide the foliage with a lemony smell when crushed. A few other *Acronychia* species are edible but have smaller fruit and are not usually cultivated. These include *A. oblongifolia* and *A. vestita*.

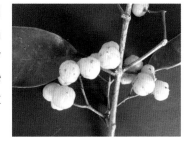

Lemon aspens can be eaten raw, but due to their tart taste, are often used in condiments and jams. They contain the polyphenols caffeic, chlorogenic, ferulic and p-coumaric acids, and flavonoids kaempferol and quercetin (Konczak *et al.* 2009). They also provide vitamins B9 (folate) and E, magnesium, manganese and zinc. The phytochemicals in lemon aspens will most likely provide important antioxidant and other health benefits when eaten. Kaempferol and quercetin contribute to reducing inflammation by inhibiting the activation of the protein NF-kB. Chlorogenic, ferulic and p-couramic acids enhance the body's ability to remove carcinogens (Napier 1998).

Lemon myrtle (*Backhousia citriodora*) is a tree that orginates from rainforests of Queensland. It is now grown commercially in several locations along the east coast of Australia. The lemon-scented leaves are infused in hot water to make a tea, and its essential oils are also considered valuable. Lemon myrtle leaf extract inhibits the intestinal enzyme alpha-glucosidase, thereby potentially slowing the absorption of glucose from our food and helping to keep blood glucose levels low (Konczak *et al*. 2012).

The leaves contain ellagic acid and the flavonoids hesperetin, myricetin and quercetin (Konczak *et al*. 2009; 2012). Research from commonly cultivated fruit and vegetables indicate that these phytochemicals are important antioxidants, provide anti-inflammatory and detoxification benefits, and potentially reduce angiogenesis, that is they inhibit the formation of blood vessels around tumours. Ellagic acid found in berries such as strawberries, helps detoxify carcinogens by enhancing phase 2 detoxification enzyme activities and activates the protein p53, promoting the death of cancer cells (Sakulnarmrat 2012; Riaz *et al*. 2017). These phytochemicals probably provide many of the same benefits through lemon myrtle tea.

Lilly pillies, riberries and water apples (*Syzygium* species) are commonly eaten fruits of rainforest trees. They are related to anise myrtle (*Syzygium anisatum*) described above, and the Indonesian tree that produces cloves, which are the dried flower buds of *Syzygium aromaticum*. The related *Syzygium cumini*, called jambolan, from South East Asia produces edible juicy fruit traditionally used in India for relieving cold symptoms, rashes and helping with diabetes (Ayyanar & Subash-Babu 2012). The dark purple fruit of jambolan contain high levels of anthocyanins, especially delphinidin and petunidin (Bhagwat & Haytowitz 2015).

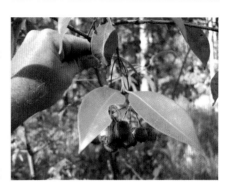

The Australian Syzygiums, *S. australe* (lilly pilly) and *S. luehmannii* (riberry), both widespread along the east coast, have been shown to have good antioxidant properties (Konczak *et al.* 2009; Jamieson *et al.* 2014). Riberries are known to contain the anthocyanin cyanidin, providing the purple fruit colour, and also kaempferol, myricetin and quercetin (Konczak *et al.* 2010; Konczak 2015). *Syzygium paniculatum* (magenta lilly pilly) from New South Wales rainforests also contains anthocyanins, plus chlorogenic and gallic acids (Vuong *et al.* 2014). The closely related *Eugenia reinwardtiana* (Cedar Bay cherry) has particularly sweet red fruit. It has chlorogenic and gallic acids, the anthocyanin cyanidin, proanthocyanins and catechins (Bhagwat & Haytowitz 2015; Konczak 2015). While all Syzygiums are likely to contain a range of vitamins, tests show water apple (*S. aqueum*) contains vitamins B1 and C.

The antioxidant properties of lilly pillies and their close relatives suggest that they can provide an important, healthy contribution to a diet. Chlorogenic acid stimulates our cells to produce the strong antioxidant, glutathione. Chlorogenic acid contributes to reducing the oxidation of LDL 'bad' cholesterol and enhances the body's ability to remove carcinogens (Napier 1998; Butt & Sultan 2011).

The presence of anthocyanins, confirmed in several species, will likely provide anti-inflammatory benefits. Anthocyanins in general can also help reduce the risk of developing cardiovascular disease, some cancers and dementia (Chen *et al.* 2006).

A word of caution. The related *Rhodomyrtus macrocarpa* (finger cherry) from north Queensland has fruit that closely resemble the lilly pilly group. Eating the fruit of finger cherry has caused people to go permanently blind and has even caused some deaths (McKenzie 2012). The mechanism has not yet been determined and may be due to a fungus that grows on the fruit, or some aspect of the fruit itself. Therefore careful identification is essential, so that lilly pilly fruit should be sourced from a reputable supplier.

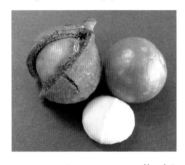

Macadamia nuts (*Macadamia* species) are Australia's most well-known bush food. There are four species of macadamia trees and a further three tropical Australian trees were once considered *Macadamia* species but are now in a separate genus called *Lasjia*. Only *M. integrifolia* and *M. tetraphylla* have edible nuts and horticultural crops of macadamia nuts are cultivars of, and hybrids between, those two species. The Macadamia Conservation Trust contribute to the long term preservation of wild populations. Macadamia nuts are cultivated across eastern Australia and in subtropical regions of the world. They contain the phytosterols, campesterol and beta-sitosterol. They also have a high content of healthy monounsaturated fats, especially oleic and palmitoleic acids. Regular consumption of macadamia nuts helps thin the blood, reduce inflammation and maintain a healthy balance between LDL 'bad' cholesterol and HDL 'good' cholesterol (Munro & Garg 2008). Greater details on macadamia nuts are provided in Chapter 15.

Native cucumber, or native melon (*Cucumis melo* subspecies *agrestis*) is reported to be edible once the fruit ripens, losing its green colour (Latz 1995). It is thought that this is the native cucumber the Australian explorer John Stuart described eating to relieve his scurvy in 1862 (Traynor & Breen 2010). Native cucumber is a small fruited subspecies of the widespread cucumber and melon plants, including rock melons (*Cucumis melo*). It is likely to contain many of the phytochemicals found in melons, including beta-carotene, lutein, a range of flavonoids and vitamin C. These phytochemicals in melons have been found to have antioxidant properties (Arora *et al.* 2011).

Native ginger (*Alpinia caerulea*) grows within rainforests, on creek banks and in wet euca- 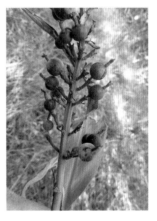 lypt forests along the east coast of Australia, from north of Sydney to Cape York Peninsula. There are four other *Alpinia* species native to Australia, although it is not known whether they are edible. The stem and leaves of native ginger are larger than common ginger (*Zingiber officinale*), and it is more closely related to galangal (*Alpinia galanga*). The thin blue flesh around the seed of native ginger is said to be edible, as are the tips of young rhizomes (roots) when chopped and cooked (Cribb & Cribb 1988). A phytochemical in the fruit called zerumin A has been found to provide anti-angiogenic properties in a laboratory study. That is, it inhibits the formation of new blood vessels, and this may be a way to inhibit or starve the growth of tumours (He *et al.* 2012). The related *Pleuranthodium racemigerum*, which is probably not edible, contains cuminoids that strongly inhibit production of the inflammatory prostaglandin E2 (Wohlmuth 2008); and native ginger may have similar compounds. Given the substantial health benefits provided by other plants in the ginger family, native ginger probably provides a wealth of beneficial phytochemicals. Research into the health benefits of its phytochemicals is likely to be very worthwhile.

Native mint (*Mentha australis*) contains chlorogenic, gallic and rosmarinic acids, and the flavanoids apigenin, hesperetin and naringenin. These phytochemicals provide native mint with an antioxidant potential similar to spearmint (Tang *et al.* 2016).

Native pepper bushes (*Tasmannia* species) are a group of attractive shrubs that grow naturally from Tasmania to north Queensland. They are typically found in rainforest, wet eucalypt forests and forest regrowth. The main species cultivated

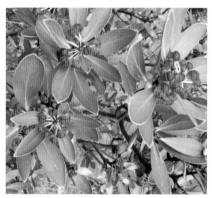

for their peppery spice are *Tasmannia lanceolata* (also called Tasmanian pepper or mountain pepper) and *T. stipitata* (also called Dorrigo pepper). The pepper flavouring is derived from both the leaves and dried fruit.

The terpene oil polygodial provides the peppery taste, and repels herbivores, probably helping the plants establish in regrowth (Read & Menary 2000). It also provides antimicrobial and antioxidant properties. Both the leaves and fruit contain the anthocyanin cyanidin (with very high levels in the fruit), chlorogenic acid and quercetin (Konczak *et al.* 2009).

Tasmanian pepper leaves have a very high antioxidant capacity (Konczak *et al.* 2009). Chlorogenic acid, cyanidin and quercetin are phytochemicals known to provide strong antioxidant and anti-inflammatory benefits, and to help reduce the development of cancer by enhancing the body's ability to remove carcinogens

(Konczak *et al.* 2009; Napier 1998). Anthocyanins from blueberries enhance mental performance and possibly provide the same benefit when consumed in native pepper bush.

Native turmeric (*Curcuma australasica*) is an attractive flowering ginger-like plant from Cape York Peninsula, which is closely related to the Indian spice turmeric (*Curcuma longa*). Native turmeric is reported to be edible after roasting (Cribb & Cribb 1988) and research into the edibility and health benefits of this turmeric should be a priority. It contains the phytochemical zederone, which inhib-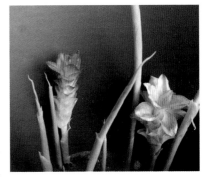its the inflammation-causing prostaglandin E2 in laboratory tests (Wohlmuth 2008).

Noni (*Morinda citrifolia*) is a tree that grows in coastal areas across northern Australia, from central Queensland to the Kimberley. It also grows naturally in many Pacific Islands, including Hawaii. As it has a reputation in several Pacific Island cultures as a food and medicine, there has been quite a bit of research into its phytochemicals. Noni fruit juice contains the flavonoids kaempferol and quercetin, and another polyphenol called scopoletin which has shown anti-inflammatory and anti-cancer properties in a laboratory trial (Nitteranon *et al.* 2011). Noni fruit also contain vitamin C and the minerals calcium and magnesium (Lim 2012c).

The few small human trials on the effect of noni juice, or extracts, in cancer patients have found evidence of decreased pain and reduced free radical levels, but no clear effect on tumours (Brown 2012). Studies suggest noni fruit can stimulate mammal immune systems by increasing the production of a type of cytokine called interferon gamma (IFN-γ; Palu *et al.* 2008).

A 30 day trial with 285 heavy smokers demonstrated that noni juice reduced the levels of free radicals, superoxide anion and lipid hydroperoxide, in their blood (Wang *et al.* 2009). Potential side effects of noni fruit and juice include nausea, possibly from the pungent smell of the fruit! The high concentration of potassium has led to advice that patients with kidney, heart or liver problems may need to avoid noni juice (Brown 2012).

Pepper vines are a group of Australian rainforest climbers closely related to the culinary black pepper, *Piper nigrum. Piper hederaceum* (previously called *P. novae-hollandiae*) has fruit that are reported to be edible when ground (Haslam & Hauser 2004). It grows in rainforest from New South Wales to north Queensland. *Piper macropiper* (previously called *P. rothianum*) also has fruit reported to be edible (Cooper & Cooper 1994) and grows in north Queensland rainforest, New Guinea and South East Asia. Cautious identification is needed, and native peppers should be sourced from a reputable supplier, as there are several other species of *Piper* in Australia as well as other similar looking vines that may not be edible, and some may be posionous.

The phytochemistry of Australian pepper vines is not known but it is intriguing to think that they may have similar health benefits to black pepper, such as reducing the inflammation of arthritis and helping reduce the risk of developing dementia (Aggarwal & Yost 2011). Black pepper also has antimicrobial properties (Butt *et al.* 2013).

Pigface, *Carpobrotus aequilaterus, C. edulis, C. glaucescens, C. modestus, C. rossii* and *C. virescens* grow on dunes along Australian beaches, from Mackay southwards around southern Australia and up to Exmouth in Western Australia. The red fruit are edible raw and have a salty taste. Research into three of the species present in Tasmania, *Carpobrotus aequilaterus, C. edulis* and *C. rossii*, found high antioxidant properties in plant juice

(Vennavaram 2007). They contain the flavonoid rutin (a variant of quercetin), gallic acid and vitamin C.

Pindan walnut (*Terminalia cunninghamii*), also known as the Kalumburu almond, is a tree that grows naturally in the Kimberley region of north Western Australia. The seed, exposed after removing the flesh and cracking the outer shell, is an important native food traditionally used by Aboriginal people of the Kimberley region (Zhong *et al.* 2017). Recent analyses of the nutritional qualities of Pindan walnut have found them to be high in protein and minerals such as magnesium and potassium (Zhong *et al.* 2017). They have levels of polyphenols, halfway between macadamia and standard walnuts, and good antioxidant properties (Zhong *et al.* 2017).

Purslane (*Portulaca oleracea*), also known as pigweed, is small semi-succulent herb that establishes as a weed of gardens, and is native across large regions of Australia and elswhere around the world. Both the leaves and seeds are edible and are an excellent source of the omega 3 fat, alpha-linolenic acid (ALA), which helps reduce inflammation. The seeds contain 34% ALA and 27% omega 6 linoleic acid (Brown *et al.* 1985). A gram of fresh leaves supplies around 1 to 1.5 mg of ALA (Liu *et al.* 2000). Purslane also contains vitamins C and E, and beta-carotene, providing good antioxidant capacity (Liu *et al.* 2000).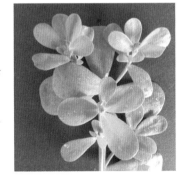

Note that the leaves have a fairly high concentration of oxalic acid (oxalates), as do some other vegetables such as spinach. Oxalates can bind to some minerals, making them harder to absorb. This includes calcium, and kidney stones are calcium oxalate. People with kidney problems, or suceptible to kidney stones, should not eat too much, if any, purslane. Steaming or boiling leaves can reduce oxalates a little.

Quandong, red (*Santalum accuminatum*) is a small tree or shrub that grows in dry areas across much of the Australian continent, and is most abundant in South Australia and southern Western Australia. It is not related to the blue quandong (*Elaeocarpus grandis*), which is a rainforest tree with fruit containing a thin outer fleshy layer that is reported to also be edible (Cribb & Cribb 1988). A laboratory trial found that red quandong extract protected cells from oxidative damage from hydrogen peroxide to a greater extent than blueberries (Sakulnarmrat *et al.* 2015). The red quandong fruit contains the anthocyanin cyanidin 3-glucoside, plus chlorogenic acid and quercetin (Konczak *et al.* 2012).

Raspberries are a familiar fruit with several species native to Australia, such as *Rubus parviflorus* and *R. queenslandicus*. Asian 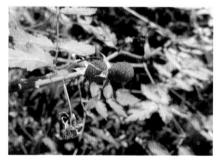 and European blackberries and raspberries have become weeds in some parts of Australia. Australian raspberries are some of the sweetest bush foods. They likely contain a range of the healthy flavonoids, especially anthocyanins, which are found in cultivated raspberries. These compounds are probably present in high concentrations given that wild plants have to produce abundant phytochemicals to protect themselves. The phytochemicals in cultivated raspberries can reduce oxidation of fats and provide some inhibition of the inflammatory-causing enzyme COX-2, as well as hinder the growth of tumour cells cultured in the laboratory (Bowen-Forbes *et al.* 2010).

Warragul greens (*Tetragonia tetragonoides*) are the edible leaves, often steamed before eating, of a large herb. It is native to Australia, New Zealand and a variety of South East Asian countries, and is also known as New Zealand spinach. Warragul greens have a reputation for being useful for relieving stomach problems, including ulcers (Ko *et al.* 2017). The leaves contain beta-carotene, ferulic acid, lutein, neoxanthin, violaxanthin, plus vitamin C and the omega 3 fat ALA (Cambie 1988; de Azevedo-Meleiro & Rodriguez-Amaya 2005; Duke 2016). Compounds distilled from the leaves show anti-inflammatory properties, resulting from the inhibition of the inflammation-promoting protein NF-kB (Ko *et al.* 2017). The beta-carotene and lutein in the leaves of Warragul greens would likely provide important anti-oxidant protection to our eyes.

Water spinach (*Ipomoea aquatica*) is a trailing large leaved herb related to morning glory. It grows in wetlands across northern Australia. Kang kong is the name given to this plant in South East Asia and it is sold in Australia as a vegetable that is typically steamed prior to eating. It spreads vigorously in the garden, so needs containment, but is sensitive to frost.

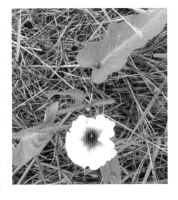

Water spinach provides the flavonoids quercetin and kaempferol, and alpha- and beta-carotene (Cribb & Cribb 1990; Lako *et al.* 2007). It also contains vitamins B1, B2, B3, C and E, plus various minerals including magnesium and zinc (Duke 2016). Based on these phytochemicals, we would expect water spinach to provide useful antioxidant and anti-inflammatory benefits.

Wattle seeds. Various species of *Acacia*, but not all, have seeds that can be ground into a flour, cooked and eaten (Latz 1995). The fats in wattle seeds are typically dominated by the omega 6 linoleic acid. However, several wattles of northern Australia contain fairly high amounts (32-56%) of oleic acid, the healthy monounsaturated omega 9 fat found in olive oil: *Acacia adsurgens, A. cowleana, A. crassicarpa, A. ligulata, A. oswaldii, A. sericophylla* (previously called *A. coriacea*), *A. tetragonophylla* and *A. tenuissima* (Brown *et al.* 1987). Oleic acid has been found to help lower blood pressure (Teres *et al.* 2008). Laboratory animal studies indicate oleic acid, taken from olive oil, can promote the death of cancer cells (Menendez *et al.* 2005).

Wattle seeds contain the polyphenols caffeic, ferulic and gallic acids and catechin (Ee *et al.* 2011). These phytochemicals have strong antioxidant properties and ferulic acid can enhance the body's ability to remove carcinogens (Napier 1998). Roasting seeds of the wattle *Acacia victoriae*, has been found to increase the availability and antioxidant actions of several phytochemicals contained in the seed (Ee *et al.* 2011). Wattle seeds also have good amounts of fibre, plus vitamins B1, B3, B6, B9 (folate) and E, and minerals such as calcium, magnesium and selenium (FSANZ 2013).

Chapter 17
Concluding thoughts

Plants are exceptional chemists and their pharmacy provides us with an enormous number of healthy compounds. Our health receives a boost when eating at least two serves of fruit and five to six serves of vegetables a day, as well as drinking tea and coffee, and eating herbs and spices. Some people recommend eating even more plants daily. An example of a serve of fruit is an apple, a banana, an orange or a cup (250 mL) of chopped fruit. A serve of vegetables is a cup of uncooked salad plants or half a cup of cooked vegetables.

To get the most out of plants, it is important to eat a wide range of fruit, vegetables, herbs and spices, providing a kaleidoscope of colour. This provides an abundance of phytochemicals and allows synergies between them. Including less commonly cultivated plants in our diet provides variety and probably some novel phytochemical combinations. A Spanish survey found that 419 different species of wild plants are consumed in the country (Tardio *et al.* 2006). People on the Greek island of Ikaria include over 150 wild vegetables and herbs in their diet (Buettner 2015). Australia has a great range of edible native bush food plants that can provide health benefits, and show great potential as regular elements of our diet.

How plants are grown and stored affects their phytochemical levels. Many phytochemicals are made by plants to deal with stressful conditions. Plants grown organically, that is without artificial pesticides or synthetic fertilsers, tend to have greater concentrations of phytochemicals than conventionally cultivated crops. In the absence of pesticides, plants produce phytochemicals to defend themselves. High levels of nitrogen and phosphorus fertilisation can reduce phytochemicals in some plants, although nitrogen fertilising has been found to increase the concentration of lutein and zeaxanthin in corn (Giordano *et al.* 2018). High levels of organic matter in the soil also promote phytochemicals. Most Australians, indeed most people in developed countries, obtain the majority of their phytochemicals from conventially grown produce. Keeping the amount of pesticides and artificial fertilisers used on crops to a minimum, and increasing soil organic matter, would likely increase the phytochemical content in conventially grown produce, thereby contributing to the health of the community.

The development of efficient and easy to use technology to test phytochemical content of produce would help growers refine growing techniques to enhance phytochemical concentrations and perhaps certify the phytochemical content of their produce. Information about the phytochemical concentrations in batches of fruit and vegetables could enhance consumer awareness and allow phytochemical content to be a factor in our food choices. However, we shouldn't become obsessed with individual phytochemicals, but instead aim to consume good levels of a diversity of them by eating a broad range of plants.

How plants are prepared for eating affects the abundance, structure and availability of phytochemicals. Some phytochemicals are best absorbed when eaten with fats, such as olive oil. This includes beta-carotene in carrots, curcumin in turmeric, lutein in spinach and lycopene in tomatoes. Cooking is useful for increasing the availability of some phytochemicals, especially the carotenoids beta-carotene in carrots and lycopene in tomatoes. This is because cooking helps release these phytochemicals from their storage compartments within plant cells. In contrast, broccoli, cabbages and cauliflower should only be steamed briefly, because heat damages the enzyme that activates their health-promoting phytochemicals. Garlic and onions require a few minutes to sit between chopping and cooking, to allow their sulphur compounds to convert to an active form. Vitamin C is also damaged by heat.

Cooking plants by submerging in hot water for long periods can leach phytochemicals into the water. This is the aim in tea production, but it is better to briefly steam most vegetables, or only boil quickly, to retain their full phytochemical content.

Our society's apparent obsession with perfect-looking food was highlighted in the 2017 and 2018 ABC television documentary series *War on Waste*. It showed the waste of perfectly good bananas that are thrown away because they do not match a pre-determined size and shape. North Queensland banana growers, Krista and Robert Watkins of Natural Evolution Foods, are helping reduce this waste by making banana flour and other products from green bananas, including those that don't meet the standard size and shape. They are also making flour from excess sweet potatoes.

The absence of minor blemishes on fruit and vegetables in many shops is another issue that should raise questions about how many artificial chemicals farmers are forced to spray onto crops. Perhaps as a community we can become more focused on the nutritional content, including phytochemicals, of our fruit and vegetables, rather than their surface appearance.

Hopefully in the near future, people will discuss phytochemicals as commonly as vitamins and minerals are discussed today, and include them in their decisions about cultivation techniques and food purchase choices.

Table 17.1 provides a summary of some of the plausible health benefits from key phytochemicals, and example plants containing them.

Happy feasting on phytochemicals!

Table 17.1. Summary of the plausible health benefits of phyto-chemicals, and example plants providing those phytochemicals

Health issue	Phytochemicals contributing to health benefits	Plants to eat that contain these phytochemicals
Cardiovascular health: Balance cholesterol levels and reduce oxidation damage to LDLs and blood vessels	Anthocyanins, beta-carotene, beta-sitosterol, catechins, curcumin, lycopene, oleocanthal and additional polyphenols	Avocados, blueberries, carrots, macadamia nuts, olive oil, pomegranate, strawberries, tea, tomatoes and turmeric
Cardiovascular health: Maintain healthy blood pressure	Betalains, catechins, piperine, quercetin, as well as nitrates	Beetroot, citrus, dark chocolate, onions, pepper and tea
Enhance detoxification	Galangin, kaempferol, limonene, naringenin, sulforaphane and tangeretin	Broccoli, cabbage, citrus - especially grapefruit, galangal and tea
Help the body resist the development of cancer	Allicin, curcumin, ellagic acid, epigallocatechin-3-gallate, gingerol, isoflavones, limonene, lycopene, naringenin, PEITC, resveratrol, sulforaphane and tangeretin	Blueberries, broccoli, cabbage, citrus, garlic, ginger, grapes, green tea, onions, soybeans, strawberries, tomatoes and turmeric
Lower inflammation and inflammatory pain	Allicin, curcumin, eugenol, gingerol, kaempferol, oleocanthal, additional polyphenols and sulforaphane	Apples, broccoli, cherries, cloves, garlic, gotu kola, ginger, olive oil, onions and turmeric

Table 2.1 *continued...*

Health issue	Phytochemicals contributing to health benefits	Plants to eat that contain these phytochemicals
Maintain and enhance mental performance and help relieve anxiety and depression	Anthocyanins, caffeine, curcumin, gingerol, lutein, omega 3 ALA, resveratrol and sulforaphane	Blueberries, broccoli, cabbage, dark chocolate, flax seed, ginger, olive oil, raspberries, sage, spinach and turmeric
Maintain a healthy weight	Anthocyanins, catechins, ellagitannins, methylhydroxychalcone and naringenin	Blackberries, blueberries, cinnamon, grapefruit, strawberries and tea
Promote eye health	Beta-carotene, lutein and zeaxanthin	Carrots, corn, kale, mustard greens and spinach
Promote healthy gut microbiota	Catechins and other flavonoids and oligosaccharides.	Dark chocolate, garlic, onions and tea
Reduce hay fever allergy symptoms	Hesperetin and quercetin	Citrus and onions

References

Abuznait, A. H., Qosa, H., Busnena, B. A., El Sayed, K. A., & Kaddoumi, A. (2013). Olive-oil-derived oleocanthal enhances β-amyloid clearance as a potential neuroprotective mechanism against Alzheimer's disease: in vitro and in vivo studies. ACS chemical neuroscience, 4(6), 973-982.

Ackermann, R. T., Mulrow, C. D., Ramirez, G., Gardner, C. D., Morbidoni, L., & Lawrence, V. A. (2001). Garlic shows promise for improving some cardiovascular risk factors. Archives of internal medicine, 161(6), 813-824.

Adamafio, N. A. (2013). Theobromine toxicity and remediation of cocoa by-products: an overview. Journal of Biological Sciences, 13(7), 570-576.

Adams N. (2014). Healthy Vision. Prevent and reverse eye disease through better nutrition. Lyons Press, Montana.

Aggarwal, B. B., & Shishodia, S. (2004). Suppression of the Nuclear Factor-κB Activation Pathway by Spice-Derived Phytochemicals: Reasoning for Seasoning. Annals of the New York Academy of Sciences, 1030(1), 434-441.

Agarwal, K. A., Tripathi, C. D., Agarwal, B. B., & Saluja, S. (2011). Efficacy of turmeric (curcumin) in pain and postoperative fatigue after laparoscopic cholecystectomy: a double-blind, randomized placebo-controlled study. Surgical endoscopy, 25(12), 3805-3810.

Agati, G., Stefano, G., Biricolti, S., & Tattini, M. (2009). Mesophyll distribution of 'antioxidant'flavonoid glycosides in Ligustrum vulgare leaves under contrasting sunlight irradiance. Annals of Botany, 104(5), 853-861.

Aggarwal, B. B., & Yost, D. (2011). Healing Spices: How to Use 50 Everyday and Exotic Spices to Boost Health and Beat Disease. Sterling Publishing Company.

Aggarwal, B., Prasad, S., Reuter, S., Kannappan, R., R Yadav, V., Park, B., ... & Prasad, S. (2011). Identification of novel anti-inflammatory agents from Ayurvedic medicine for prevention of chronic diseases:'reverse pharmacology' and 'bedside to bench' approach. Current drug targets, 12(11), 1595-1653.

Aggarwal, B. B., Gupta, S. C., & Sung, B. (2013). Curcumin: an orally bioavailable blocker of TNF and other pro-inflammatory biomarkers. British journal of pharmacology, 169(8), 1672-1692.

Ahuja, K. D., Robertson, I. K., Geraghty, D. P., & Ball, M. J. (2006). Effects of chili consumption on postprandial glucose, insulin, and energy metabolism−. The American journal of clinical nutrition, 84(1), 63-69.

AIHW (2017). Cardiovascular health compendium. Australian Institute of Health and Welfare. Australian Government.

Al-Youssef, H. M., & Hassan, W. H. (2017). Chemical constituents of Carissa edulis Vahl. Arabian Journal of Chemistry, 10(1), 109-113.

Ale-Agha N, Goy C, Jakobs P, Spyridopoulos I, Gonnissen S, Dyballa-Rukes N, et al. (2018) CDKN1B/p27 is localized in mitochondria and improves respiration-dependent processes in the cardiovascular system—New mode of action for caffeine. PLoS Biol 16(6): e2004408.

Alharbi, M. H., Lamport, D. J., Dodd, G. F., Saunders, C., Harkness, L., Butler, L. T., & Spencer, J. P. (2016). Flavonoid-rich orange juice is associated with acute improvements in cognitive function in healthy middle-aged males. European journal of nutrition, 55(6), 2021-2029.

Ali, R., Barnes, I., Kan, S. W., & Beral, V. (2010). Cancer incidence in British Indians and British whites in Leicester, 2001–2006. British journal of cancer, 103(1), 143.

Ali, T., Shakir, F., & Morton, J. (2012). Curcumin and inflammatory bowel disease: biological mechanisms and clinical implication. Digestion, 85(4), 249-255.

Allman, M. A., Pena, M. M., & Pang, D. (1995). Supplementation with flaxseed oil versus sunflowerseed oil in healthy young men consuming a low fat diet: effects on platelet composition and function. European journal of clinical nutrition, 49(3), 169-178.

Altman, R. D., & Marcussen, K. C. (2001). Effects of a ginger extract on knee pain in patients with osteoarthritis. Arthritis & Rheumatology, 44(11), 2531-2538.

Alvarez-Suarez, J. M., Giampieri, F., Tulipani, S., Casoli, T., Di Stefano, G., González-Paramás, A. M., ... & Bompadre, S. (2014). One-month strawberry-rich anthocyanin supplementation ameliorates cardiovascular risk, oxidative stress markers and platelet activation in humans. The Journal of nutritional biochemistry, 25(3), 289-294.

Amiot, M. J., Riva, C., & Vinet, A. (2016). Effects of dietary polyphenols on metabolic syndrome features in humans: a systematic review. Obesity Reviews, 17(7), 573-586.

Anderson, R. A., Zhan, Z., Luo, R., Guo, X., Guo, Q., Zhou, J., ... & Stoecker, B. J. (2016). Cinnamon extract lowers glucose, insulin and cholesterol in people with elevated serum glucose. Journal of traditional and complementary medicine, 6(4), 332-336.

wAnand, P., Kunnumakara, A. B., Sundaram, C., Harikumar, K. B., Tharakan, S. T., Lai, O. S., ... & Aggarwal, B. B. (2008). Cancer is a preventable disease that requires major lifestyle changes. Pharmaceutical research, 25(9), 2097-2116.

Appel, L. J., Moore, T. J., Obarzanek, E., Vollmer, W. M., Svetkey, L. P., Sacks, F. M., ... & Lin, P. H. (1997). A clinical trial of the effects of dietary patterns on blood pressure. New England Journal of Medicine, 336(16), 1117-1124.

Arora, R., Kaur, M., & Gill, N. S. (2011). Antioxidant activity and pharmacological evaluation of Cucumis melo var. agrestis methanolic seed extract. Research journal of phytochemistry, 5(3), 146-155.

Atanasov, A. G., Waltenberger, B., Pferschy-Wenzig, E. M., Linder, T., Wawrosch, C., Uhrin, P., ... & Rollinger, J. M. (2015). Discovery and resupply of pharmacologically active plant-derived natural products: A review. Biotechnology advances, 33(8), 1582-1614.

Austin, D. F. (2007). Water spinach (Ipomoea aquatica, Convolvulaceae): a food gone wild. Ethnobotany Research and Applications, 5, 123-146.

Aviram, M., Rosenblat, M., Gaitini, D., Nitecki, S., Hoffman, A., Dornfeld, L., ... & Hayek, T. (2004). Pomegranate juice consumption for 3 years by patients with carotid artery stenosis reduces common carotid intima-media thickness, blood pressure and LDL oxidation. Clinical Nutrition, 23(3), 423-433.

Avoseh, O., Oyedeji, O., Rungqu, P., Nkeh-Chungag, B., & Oyedeji, A. (2015). Cymbopogon species; ethnopharmacology, phytochemistry and the pharmacological importance. Molecules, 20(5), 7438-7453.

Ayyanar, M., & Subash-Babu, P. (2012). Syzygium cumini (L.) Skeels: A review of its phytochemical constituents and traditional uses. Asian Pacific journal of tropical biomedicine, 2(3), 240-246.

Azam, S., Hadi, N., Khan, N. U., & Hadi, S. M. (2004). Prooxidant property of green tea polyphenols epicatechin and epigallocatechin-3-gallate: implications for anticancer properties. Toxicology in vitro, 18(5), 555-561.

Baliga, M. S., Pai, R. J., Bhat, H. P., Palatty, P. L., & Boloor, R. (2011). Chemistry and medicinal properties of the Bakul (Mimusops elengi Linn): A review. Food research international, 44(7), 1823-1829.

Banerjee, S., Ji, C., Mayfield, J. E., Goel, A., Xiao, J., Dixon, J. E., & Guo, X. (2018). Ancient drug curcumin impedes 26S proteasome activity by direct inhibition of dual-specificity tyrosine-regulated kinase 2. Proceedings of the National Academy of Sciences, 201806797.

Barański, M., Średnicka-Tober, D., Volakakis, N., Seal, C., Sanderson, R., Stewart, G. B., ... & Gromadzka-Ostrowska, J. (2014). Higher antioxidant and lower cadmium concentrations and lower incidence of pesticide residues in organically grown crops: a systematic literature review and meta-analyses. British Journal of Nutrition, 112(05), 794-811.

Baslam, M., Garmendia, I., & Goicoechea, N. (2011). Arbuscular mycorrhizal fungi (AMF) improved growth and nutritional quality of greenhouse-grown lettuce. Journal of agricultural and food chemistry, 59(10), 5504-5515.

Baspinar, B., Eskici, G., & Ozcelik, A. O. (2017). How coffee affects metabolic syndrome and its components. Food & Function.

Bassiri-Jahromi, S.(2018). Punica granatum (Pomegranate) activity in health promotion and cancer prevention. Oncology Reviews, 12, 1.

Basu, A., Wilkinson, M., Penugonda, K., Simmons, B., Betts, N. M., & Lyons, T. J. (2009). Freeze-dried strawberry powder improves lipid profile and lipid peroxidation in women with metabolic syndrome: baseline and post intervention effects. Nutrition journal, 8(1), 43.

Basu, A., Sanchez, K., Leyva, M. J., Wu, M., Betts, N. M., Aston, C. E., & Lyons, T. J. (2010). Green tea supplementation affects body weight, lipids, and lipid peroxidation in obese subjects with metabolic syndrome. Journal of the American College of Nutrition, 29(1), 31-40.

Batliwala, S., Xavier, C., Liu, Y., Wu, H., & Pang, I. H. (2017). Involvement of Nrf2 in ocular diseases. Oxidative medicine and cellular longevity, 2017.

Beauchamp, G. K., Keast, R. S., Morel, D., Lin, J., Pika, J., Han, Q., ... & Breslin, P. A. (2005). Phytochemistry: ibuprofen-like activity in extra-virgin olive oil. Nature, 437(7055), 45-46.

Béliveau R. (2018). Better understanding of the anticancer effect of curcuma. Translation from Le Journal de Montreal, 3 September 2018. Accessed: https://www.richardbeliveau.org/wp-content/uploads/630-Curcum-in-and-proteasome-2018-09-03-CompressedSecured.pdf

Béliveau R. and Gingras D. (2014) Preventing Cancer. The complete wellness guide to reducing the risks of cancer and helping recovery. Les Editions due Trecarre, Montreal, Quebec, Canada.

Béliveau, R., & Gingras, D. (2017). Foods to Fight Cancer: What to Eat to Reduce Your Risk. Dorling Kindersley Ltd.

Bell, P. G., Walshe, I. H., Davison, G. W., Stevenson, E., & Howatson, G. (2014). Montmorency cherries reduce the oxidative stress and inflammatory responses to repeated days high-intensity stochastic cycling. Nutrients, 6(2), 829-843.

Bellingrath, S., Rohleder, N., & Kudielka, B. M. (2013). Effort–reward-imbalance in healthy teachers is associated with higher LPS-stimulated production and lower glucocorticoid sensitivity of interleukin-6 in vitro. Biological psychology, 92(2), 403-409.

Benavides, G. A., Squadrito, G. L., Mills, R. W., Patel, H. D., Isbell, T. S., Patel, R. P., ... & Kraus, D. W. (2007). Hydrogen sulfide mediates the vasoactivity of garlic. Proceedings of the National Academy of Sciences, 104(46), 17977-17982.

Benetou, V., Orfanos, P., Lagiou, P., Trichopoulos, D., Boffetta, P., & Trichopoulou, A. (2008). Vegetables and fruits in relation to cancer risk: evidence from the Greek EPIC cohort study. Cancer Epidemiology Biomarkers & Prevention, 17(2), 387-392.

Bergquist, S. Å., Gertsson, U. E., Knuthsen, P., & Olsson, M. E. (2005). Flavonoids in baby spinach (Spinacia oleracea L.): changes during plant growth and storage. Journal of agricultural and food chemistry, 53(24), 9459-9464.

Berhow, M., Tisserat B., Kanes K., and Vandercook C. (1998). Survey of phenolic compounds produced in Citrus. United States Department of Agriculture, Technical Bulletin Number 1856.

Best, R., Lewis, D. A., & Nasser, N. (1984). The anti-ulcerogenic activity of the unripe plantain banana (Musa species). British journal of pharmacology, 82(1), 107-116.

Bevege, L. (2004). Centella asiatica: a review. Australian Journal of Medical Herbalism, 16(1), 15.

Bhagwat, S., & Haytowitz, D. B. (2015). USDA Database for the Flavonoid Content of Selected Foods Release 3.2.

Binosha, F. W., Somaratne, G., Williams, S., Goozee, K. G., Singh, H., & Martins, R. N. (2017). Diabetes and Alzheimer's Disease: Can Tea Phytochemicals Play a Role in Prevention? Journal of Alzheimer's Disease, (Preprint), 1-21.

Birtić, S., Dussort, P., Pierre, F. X., Bily, A. C., & Roller, M. (2015). Carnosic acid. Phytochemistry, 115, 9-19.

Bischoff, S. C. (2008). Quercetin: potentials in the prevention and therapy of disease. Current Opinion in Clinical Nutrition & Metabolic Care, 11(6), 733-740.

Black, C. D., Herring, M. P., Hurley, D. J., & O'Connor, P. J. (2010). Ginger (Zingiber officinale) reduces muscle pain caused by eccentric exercise. The Journal of Pain, 11(9), 894-903.

Bliddal, H., Rosetzsky, A., Schlichting, P., Weidner, M. S., Andersen, L. A., Ibfelt, H. H., ... & Barslev, J. (2000). A randomized, placebo-controlled, cross-over study of ginger extracts and ibuprofen in osteoarthritis. Osteoarthritis and Cartilage, 8(1), 9-12.

Bloch-Dano E. and Fagan T. L. (2012).'Vegetables a Biography'. The University of Chicago Press.

Block, E. (1985). The chemistry of garlic and onions. Scientific American, 252, 3,: 114-119.

Bolling, B. W., Chen, C. Y. O., McKay, D. L., & Blumberg, J. B. (2011). Tree nut phytochemicals: composition, antioxidant capacity, bioactivity, impact factors. A systematic review of almonds, Brazils, cashews, hazelnuts, macadamias, pecans, pine nuts, pistachios and walnuts. Nutrition research reviews, 24(02), 244-275.

Boonyuen, C., Wangkarn, S., Suntornwat, O., & Chaisuksant, R. (2009). Antioxidant capacity and phenolic content of Mimusops elengi fruit extract. Kasetsart J Nat Sci, 43(1), 21-27.

Borek, C. (2006). Garlic reduces dementia and heart-disease risk. The Journal of nutrition, 136(3), 810S-812S.

Bourassa, M. W., Alim, I., Bultman, S. J., & Ratan, R. R. (2016). Butyrate, neuroepigenetics and the gut microbiome: can a high fiber diet improve brain health?. Neuroscience letters, 625, 56-63.

Bovier, E. R., & Hammond, B. R. (2015). A randomized placebo-controlled study on the effects of lutein and zeaxanthin on visual processing speed in young healthy subjects. Archives of biochemistry and biophysics, 572, 54-57.

Bowen-Forbes, C. S., Zhang, Y., & Nair, M. G. (2010). Anthocyanin content, antioxidant, anti-inflammatory and anticancer properties of blackberry and raspberry fruits. Journal of food composition and analysis, 23(6), 554-560.

Boyle, G. M., D'Souza, M. M., Pierce, C. J., Adams, R. A., Cantor, A. S., Johns, J. P., Maslovskaya, L., Gordon, V. A., Reddell, P. W. & Parsons, P. G. (2014)Intralesional injection of the novel PKC activator EBC-46 rapidly ablates tumors in mouse models. PLoS One, 9(10), e108887.

Bradford, P. G., & Awad, A. B. (2007). Phytosterols as anticancer compounds. Molecular nutrition & food research, 51(2), 161-170.

Brand-Miller, J. C., & Holt, S. H. (1998). Australian Aboriginal plant foods: a consideration of their nutritional composition and health implications. Nutrition Research Reviews, 11(1), 5-23.

Braune, A., & Blaut, M. (2016). Bacterial species involved in the conversion of dietary flavonoids in the human gut. Gut microbes, 7(3), 216-234.

Bredesen, D. (2017). The End of Alzheimer's: The First Program to Prevent and Reverse Cognitive Decline. Penguin.

Brock, J. (1997). Native plants of northern Australia. Reed New Holland.

Brown, A. C. (2012). Anticancer activity of Morinda citrifolia (Noni) fruit: a review. Phytotherapy Research, 26(10), 1427-1440.

Brown, A.J. P., Roberts, D.C.K and Cherikoff V. (1985). Fatty Acids in Indigenous Australian Foods. Proceedings of the Nutrition Society of Australia, 10, 209-212.

Brown, A. J., Cherikoff, V., & Roberts, D. C. K. (1987). Fatty acid composition of seeds from the Australian Acacia species. Lipids, 22(7), 490-494.

Brown, E. J., Khodr, H., Hider, C. R., & Rice-Evans, C. A. (1998). Structural dependence of flavonoid interactions with Cu2+ ions: implications for their antioxidant properties. Biochemical Journal, 330(3), 1173-1178.

Brukner P. (2018). A Fat Lot of Good. How the experts got food and diet so wrong and what you can do to take back control of your health. Penguin Randon House Australia.

Brunetti, C., Guidi, L., Sebastiani, F., & Tattini, M. (2015). Isoprenoids and phenylpropanoids are key components of the antioxidant defense system of plants facing severe excess light stress. Environmental and Experimental Botany, 119, 54-62.

Brunning A. (2015) 'Why Does Asparagus Make Your Wee Smell? And 57 other curious food and drink questions.' Orion Books, London.

Bryan N., Zand, J. and Gottlieb, B. (2010). The Nitric Oxide (NO) Solution: How to Boost the Body's Miracle Molecule. Neogenis, Texas.

Buelna-Chontal, M., & Zazueta, C. (2013). Redox activation of Nrf2 & NF-κB: a double end sword?. Cellular signalling, 25(12), 2548-2557.

Buettner D. (2015). 'The Blue Zones solution: eating and living like the world's healthiest people.' National Geographic Society, Washington D.C.

Bullmore E. (2018). The Inflamed Mind. A Radical Approach to Depression. Simon & Schuster, London.

Burton-Freeman, B., Linares, A., Hyson, D., & Kappagoda, T. (2010). Strawberry modulates LDL oxidation and postprandial lipemia in response to high-fat meal in overweight hyperlipidemic men and women. Journal of the American College of Nutrition, 29(1), 46-54.

Butera, D., Tesoriere, L., Di Gaudio, F., Bongiorno, A., Allegra, M., Pintaudi, A. M., ... & Livrea, M. A. (2002). Antioxidant activities of Sicilian prickly pear (Opuntia ficus indica) fruit extracts and reducing properties of its betalains: betanin and indicaxanthin. Journal of agricultural and food chemistry, 50(23), 6895-6901.

Butkhup, L., & Samappito, S. (2008). An analysis on flavonoids contents in Mao Luang fruits of fifteen cultivars (Antidesma bunius), grown in northeast Thailand. Pakistan journal of biological sciences, 11(7), 996-1002.

Butt, M. S., Pasha, I., Sultan, M. T., Randhawa, M. A., Saeed, F., & Ahmed, W. (2013). Black pepper and health claims: a comprehensive treatise. Critical reviews in food science and nutrition, 53(9), 875-886.

Butt, M. S., & Sultan, M. T. (2011). Coffee and its consumption: benefits and risks. Critical reviews in food science and nutrition, 51(4), 363-373.

Bylka, W., Znajdek-Awiżeń, P., Studzińska-Sroka, E., Dańczak-Pazdrowska, A., & Brzezińska, M. (2014). Centella asiatica in dermatology: an overview. Phytotherapy research, 28(8), 1117-1124.

Caldas, A. P. S., Chaves, L. O., Silva, L. L. D., Morais, D. D. C., & Alfenas, R. D. C. G. (2017). Mechanisms Involved in the Cardioprotective Effect of Avocado Consumption: A Systematic Review. International Journal of Food Properties, (In Press).

Cambie, R. C. (1988). A New Zealand phytochemical register. Part IV. Journal of the Royal Society of New Zealand, 18(2), 137-184.

Campbell R. and Gibson J. (2017). Eat Wild Tasmanian. Fullers Publishing Hobart.

Campbell T. C. and Campbell T. M. (2006). The China study: the most comprehensive study of nutrition ever conducted and the startling implications for diet, weight loss and long-term health. BenBella Books, Inc.

Canene-Adams, K., Lindshield, B. L., Wang, S., Jeffery, E. H., Clinton, S. K., & Erdman, J. W. (2007). Combinations of tomato and broccoli enhance antitumor activity in dunning r3327-h prostate adenocarcinomas. Cancer research, 67(2), 836-843.

Cannac, M., Ferrat, L., Barboni, T., Chiaramonti, N., Morandini, F., & Pasqualini, V. (2011). Identification of flavonoids in PinusLaricio needles and changes occurring after prescribed burning. Chemoecology, 21(1), 9-17.

Cano-Marquina, A., Tarín, J. J., & Cano, A. (2013). The impact of coffee on health. Maturitas, 75(1), 7-21.

Cardona, F., Andrés-Lacueva, C., Tulipani, S., Tinahones, F. J., & Queipo-Ortuño, M. I. (2013). Benefits of polyphenols on gut microbiota and implications in human health. The Journal of nutritional biochemistry, 24(8), 1415-1422.

Carnevale, L., D'Angelosante, V., Landolfi, A., Grillea, G., Selvetella, G., Storto, M., ... & Carnevale, D. (2018). Brain MRI fiber-tracking reveals white matter alterations in hypertensive patients without damage at conventional neuroimaging. Cardiovascular research.

Carvalho, R. R., Pellizzon, C. H., Justulin, L., Felisbino, S. L., Vilegas, W., Bruni, F., ... & Hiruma-Lima, C. A. (2009). Effect of mangiferin on the development of periodontal disease: Involvement of lipoxin A 4, anti-chemotaxic action in leukocyte rolling. Chemico-biological interactions, 179(2), 344-350.

Castleman, M. (2017). The New Healing Herbs: The Essential Guide to More Than 130 of Nature's Most Potent Herbal Remedies. Rodale.

Caton, J., & Hardwick, R. (2016). Field guide to useful native plants from temperate Australia. New Holland Publishers Ltd.

Ceccarelli, N., Curadi, M., Martelloni, L., Sbrana, C., Picciarelli, P., & Giovannetti, M. (2010). Mycorrhizal colonization impacts on phenolic content and antioxidant properties of artichoke leaves and flower heads two years after field transplant. Plant and Soil, 335(1-2), 311-323.

Cerella, C., Jacob, C., Viry, E., Diederich, M., Kelkel, M., & Dicato, M. (2011). Naturally occurring organic sulfur compounds: an example of a multitasking class of phytochemicals in anti-cancer research. INTECH Open Access Publisher.

Cesco, S., Mimmo, T., Tonon, G., Tomasi, N., Pinton, R., Terzano, R., ... & Nannipieri, P. (2012). Plant-borne flavonoids released into the rhizosphere: impact on soil bio-activities related to plant nutrition. A review. Biology and Fertility of Soils, 48(2), 123-149.

Chang, S. C., Cassidy, A., Willett, W. C., Rimm, E. B., O'Reilly, E. J., & Okereke, O. I. (2016). Dietary flavonoid intake and risk of incident depression in midlife and older women−3. The American journal of clinical nutrition, 104(3), 704-714.

Chatzi, L., Apostolaki, G., Bibakis, I., Skypala, I., Bibaki-Liakou, V., Tzanakis, N., ... & Cullinan, P. (2007). Protective effect of fruits, vegetables and the Mediterranean diet on asthma and allergies among children in Crete. Thorax, 62(8), 677-683.

Chaliha, M., Williams, D., Edwards, D., Pun, S., Smyth, H., & Sultanbawa, Y. (2017). Bioactive rich extracts from Terminalia ferdinandiana by enzyme-assisted extraction: A simple food safe extraction method. Journal of Medicinal Plants Research, 11(5), 96-106.

Chandran, B., & Goel, A. (2012). A randomized, pilot study to assess the efficacy and safety of curcumin in patients with active rheumatoid arthritis. Phytotherapy research, 26(11), 1719-1725.

Chang, Q., Szegedi, S. S., O'Connor, J. C., Dantzer, R., & Kelley, K. W. (2009). Cytokine-induced sickness behavior and depression. In The neuroimmunological basis of behavior and mental disorders (pp. 145-181). Springer, Boston, MA.

Chen, P. N., Chu, S. C., Chiou, H. L., Kuo, W. H., Chiang, C. L., & Hsieh, Y. S. (2006). Mulberry anthocyanins, cyanidin 3-rutinoside and cyanidin 3-glucoside, exhibited an inhibitory effect on the migration and invasion of a human lung cancer cell line. Cancer letters, 235(2), 248-259.

Cherikoff V. (2015). Wild Foods. Looking back 60,years for clues to our future survival. New Holland Publishers, London.

Choudhary, S. P., & Tran, L. S. (2011). Phytosterols: perspectives in human nutrition and clinical therapy. Current medicinal chemistry, 18(29), 4557-4567.

Christofferson, T. (2017). 'Tripping over the Truth: How the Metabolic Theory of Cancer Is Overturning One of Medicine's Most Entrenched Paradigms.' Chelsea Green Publishing.

Clarke, J. M., Topping, D. L., Bird, A. R., Young, G. P., & Cobiac, L. (2008). Effects of high-amylose maize starch and butyrylated high-amylose maize starch on azoxymethane-induced intestinal cancer in rats. Carcinogenesis, 29(11), 2190-2194.

Clarke, K. A., Dew, T. P., Watson, R. E., Farrar, M. D., Osman, J. E., Nicolaou, A., ... & Williamson, G. (2016). Green tea catechins and their metabolites in human skin before and after exposure to ultraviolet radiation. The Journal of nutritional biochemistry, 27, 203-210.

Close, D. C., & McArthur, C. (2002). Rethinking the role of many plant phenolics– protection from photodamage not herbivores?. Oikos, 99(1), 166-172.

Cocate, P. G., Natali, A. J., de Oliveira, A., Longo, G. Z., Rita de Cássia, G. A., Maria do Carmo, G. P., ... & Hermsdorff, H. H. M. (2014). Fruit and vegetable intake and related nutrients are associated with oxidative stress markers in middle-aged men. Nutrition, 30(6), 660-665.

Cock, I. E. (2015). The medicinal properties and phytochemistry of plants of the genus Terminalia (Combretaceae). Inflammopharmacology, 23(5), 203-229.

Cock, I. E., & Mohanty, S. (2011). Evaluation of the antibacterial activity and toxicity of Terminalia ferdinandia fruit extracts. Pharmacognosy Journal, 3(20), 72-79.

Collins, D. J., Simpson, G. W., Solomon, D. H., & Spurling, T. H. (2004). James Robert Price, 1912–1999. Historical Records of Australian Science, 15(1), 95-120.

Colquhoun, D. M., Moores, D., Somerset, S. M., & Humphries, J. A. (1992). Comparison of the effects on lipoproteins and apolipoproteins of a diet high in monounsaturated fatty acids, enriched with avocado, and a high-carbohydrate diet. The American journal of clinical nutrition, 56(4), 671-677.

Cooper, W., & Cooper, W. T. (1994). Fruits of the rainforest. A Guide to Fruits in Australian Trpical Rainfrests. RD Press, Chatswood NSW.

Cooper, W., & Cooper, W. T. (2004). Fruits of the Australian tropical rainforest. Nokomis Editions.

Corbi G., Conti V., Davinelli S., Scapagnini G., Filippelli A. and Ferrar N. (2016). Dietary Phytochemicals in neuroimmunoaging: a new therapeutic possibility for humans. Frontiers in Pharmacology 7: 364.

Corzo-Martínez, M., Corzo, N., & Villamiel, M. (2007). Biological properties of onions and garlic. Trends in food science & technology, 18(12), 609-625.

Cornelis, M. C., El-Sohemy, A., Kabagambe, E. K., & Campos, H. (2006). Coffee, CYP1A2 genotype, and risk of myocardial infarction. Jama, 295(10), 1135-1141.

Costello, G., Gregory, M. and Donatiu, P. 2009. Southern Macadamia Species Recovery Plan. Report to Department of the Environment, Water, Heritage and the Arts, Canberra by Horticulture Australia Limited, Sydney.

Covas, M. I. (2007). Olive oil and the cardiovascular system. Pharmacological Research, 55(3), 175-186.

Covas, M. I., Nyyssönen, K., Poulsen, H. E., Kaikkonen, J., Zunft, H. J. F., Kiesewetter, H., ... & Nascetti, S. (2006). The effect of polyphenols in olive oil on heart disease risk factors: a randomized trial. Annals of internal medicine, 145(5), 333-341.

Craig, W. J. (1997). Phytochemicals: guardians of our health. Journal of the American Dietetic Association, 97(10), S199-S204.

Cribb A. B. and Cribb J. W. (1988). 'Wild Medicine in Australia.' Angus and Roberts North Ryde, Sydney.

Cribb A. B. and Cribb J. W. (1990). 'Wild Food in Australia.' Second edition. Angus and Roberts North Ryde, Sydney.

Croft, K. D. (2016). Dietary polyphenols: Antioxidants or not?. Archives of biochemistry and biophysics, 595, 120-124.

Crozier, T. W., Stalmach, A., Lean, M. E., & Crozier, A. (2012). Espresso coffees, caffeine and chlorogenic acid intake: potential health implications. Food & function, 3(1), 30-33.

Daily, J. W., Yang, M., & Park, S. (2016). Efficacy of turmeric extracts and curcumin for alleviating the symptoms of joint arthritis: a systematic review and meta-analysis of randomized clinical trials. Journal of medicinal food, 19(8), 717-729.

Das, K., & Roychoudhury, A. (2014). Reactive oxygen species (ROS) and response of antioxidants as ROS-scavengers during environmental stress in plants. Frontiers in Environmental Science, 2, 53.

Davidson, M. H., Maki, K. C., Dicklin, M. R., Feinstein, S. B., Witchger, M., Bell, M., ... & Aviram, M. (2009). Effects of consumption of pomegranate juice on carotid intima–media thickness in men and women at moderate risk for coronary heart disease. American Journal of Cardiology, 104(7), 936-942.

Davis, D. R. (2009). Declining fruit and vegetable nutrient composition: What is the evidence?. HortScience, 44(1), 15-19.

De Alzaa, F., Guillaume, C. & Ravetti, L. (2018). Evaluation of Chemical and Physical Changes in Different Commercial Oils during Heating. Acta Scientific Nutritional Health, 2 (6), 02-11.

de Azevedo-Meleiro, C. H., & Rodriguez-Amaya, D. B. (2005). Carotenoids of endive and New Zealand spinach as affected by maturity, season and minimal processing. Journal of Food Composition and Analysis, 18(8), 845-855.

de Falco, B., Amato, M., & Lanzotti, V. (2017). Chia seeds products: an overview. Phytochemistry Reviews, 16(4), 745-760.

de Punder, K., & Pruimboom, L. (2013). The dietary intake of wheat and other cereal grains and their role in inflammation. Nutrients, 5(3), 771-787.

Del Rio, D., Rodriguez-Mateos, A., Spencer, J. P., Tognolini, M., Borges, G., & Crozier, A. (2013). Dietary (poly) phenolics in human health: structures, bioavailability, and evidence of protective effects against chronic diseases. Antioxidants & redox signaling, 18(14), 1818-1892.

de Mejia, E. G., & Ramirez-Mares, M. V. (2014). Impact of caffeine and coffee on our health. Trends in Endocrinology & Metabolism, 25(10), 489-492.

Desideri, G., Kwik-Uribe, C., Grassi, D., Necozione, S., Ghiadoni, L., Mastroiacovo, D., ... & Marini, C. (2012). Benefits in cognitive function, blood pressure, and insulin resistance through cocoa flavanol consumption in elderly subjects with mild cognitive impairment. Hypertension, HYPERTENSION AHA-112.

Devi, K. P., Malar, D. S., Nabavi, S. F., Sureda, A., Xiao, J., Nabavi, S. M., & Daglia, M. (2015). Kaempferol and inflammation: From chemistry to medicine. Pharmacological research, 99, 1-10.

Devore, E. E., Kang, J. H., Breteler, M., & Grodstein, F. (2012). Dietary intakes of berries and flavonoids in relation to cognitive decline. Annals of neurology, 72(1), 135-143.

Di Meo, F., Lemaur, V., Cornil, J., Lazzaroni, R., Duroux, J. L., Olivier, Y., & Trouillas, P. (2013). Free radical scavenging by natural polyphenols: atom versus electron transfer. The Journal of Physical Chemistry A, 117(10), 2082-2092.

Ding, H., Chin, Y. W., Kinghorn, A. D., & D'Ambrosio, S. M. (2007). Chemopreventive characteristics of avocado fruit. Seminars in cancer biology, 17: 386-394.

Djoussé, L., Folsom, A. R., Province, M. A., Hunt, S. C., & Ellison, R. C. (2003). Dietary linolenic acid and carotid atherosclerosis: the national heart, lung, and blood institute family heart study. The American journal of clinical nutrition, 77(4), 819-825.

Dod, H. S., Bhardwaj, R., Sajja, V., Weidner, G., Hobbs, G. R., Konat, G. W., ... & Beto, R. J. (2010). Effect of intensive lifestyle changes on endothelial function and on inflammatory markers of atherosclerosis. American Journal of Cardiology, 105(3), 362-367.

Domenichiello, A. F., Kitson, A. P., & Bazinet, R. P. (2015). Is docosahexaenoic acid synthesis from α-linolenic acid sufficient to supply the adult brain? Progress in lipid research, 59, 54-66.

Dong, Y., Cao, A., Shi, J., Yin, P., Wang, L., Ji, G., ... & Wu, D. (2014). Tangeretin, a citrus polymethoxyflavonoid, induces apoptosis of human gastric cancer AGS cells through extrinsic and intrinsic signaling pathways. Oncology reports, 31(4), 1788-1794.

Dorogokupla, A. C., Troitzkaia, E. G., Adilgereieva, L. K., Postolnikov, S. F., & Chekrigina, Z. P. (1973). Effect of carotene on the development of induced tumors. Zdravoor. Kazak, 10, 32-34. Cited in: Hercberg, S. (2005). The history of β-carotene and cancers: from observational to intervention studies. What lessons can be drawn for future research on polyphenols?. The American journal of clinical nutrition, 81(1), 218S-222S.

Doughman, S. D., Krupanidhi, S., & Sanjeevi, C. B. (2007). Omega-3 fatty acids for nutrition and medicine: considering microalgae oil as a vegetarian source of EPA and DHA. Current diabetes reviews, 3(3), 198.

Dreher, M. L., & Davenport, A. J. (2013). Hass avocado composition and potential health effects. Critical reviews in food science and nutrition, 53(7), 738-750.

Drewes, F. E., Smith, M. T., & Van Staden, J. (1995). The effect of a plant-derived smoke extract on the germination of light-sensitive lettuce seed. Plant Growth Regulation, 16(2), 205-209.

Duester, K. C. (2001). Avocado fruit is a rich source of beta-sitosterol. Journal of the American Dietetic Association, 101(4), 404-405.

Duke (2016). Dr. Duke's Phytochemical and Ethnobotanical Databases. U.S. Department of Agriculture, Agricultural Research Service. 1992-2016.http://phytochem.nal.usda.gov/ http://dx.doi.org/10.15482/USDA.ADC/1239279

Dutta-Roy K., Crosbie L., Gordon M. J., (2001). Effects of tomato extract on human platelet aggregation in vitro. Platelets, 12(4), 218-227.

Dyerberg, J., Bang, H. O., Stoffersen, E., Moncada, S., & Vane, J. R. (1978). Eicosapentaenoic acid and prevention of thrombosis and atherosclerosis?. The Lancet, 312(8081), 117-119.

Eberhardt, M. V., Lee, C. Y. & Liu, R. H. (2000) Antioxidant activity of fresh apples. Nature 405: 903–904.

Edirisinghe, I., Banaszewski, K., Cappozzo, J., Sandhya, K., Ellis, C. L., Tadapaneni, R., ... & Burton-Freeman, B. M. (2011). Strawberry anthocyanin and its association with postprandial inflammation and insulin. British journal of nutrition, 106(6), 913-922.

Edwards, R. L., Lyon, T., Litwin, S. E., Rabovsky, A., Symons, J. D., & Jalili, T. (2007). Quercetin reduces blood pressure in hypertensive subjects. The Journal of nutrition, 137(11), 2405-2411.

Ee, K. Y., Agboola, S., Rehman, A., & Zhao, J. (2011). Characterisation of phenolic components present in raw and roasted wattle (Acacia victoriae Bentham) seeds. Food chemistry, 129(3), 816-821.

Egert, S., Bosy-Westphal, A., Seiberl, J., Kürbitz, C., Settler, U., Plachta-Danielzik, S., ... & Wolffram, S. (2009). Quercetin reduces systolic blood pressure and plasma oxidised low-density lipoprotein concentrations in overweight subjects with a high-cardiovascular disease risk phenotype: a double-blinded, placebo-controlled cross-over study. British Journal of Nutrition, 102(7), 1065-1074.

Egner, P. A., Chen, J. G., Zarth, A. T., Ng, D. K., Wang, J. B., Kensler, K. H., ... & Fahey, J. W. (2014). Rapid and sustainable detoxication of airborne pollutants by broccoli sprout beverage: results of a randomized clinical trial in China. Cancer prevention research, 7(8), 813-823.

Elliott W. H. and Elliott D. C. (2009). Biochemistry and Molecular Biology. Fourth Edition. Oxford University Press.

Enders, G. (2015). Gut: The Inside Story of Our Body's Most Underrated Organ. Scribe Publications, Melbourne.

Esatbeyoglu, T., Wagner, A. E., Schini-Kerth, V. B., & Rimbach, G. (2015). Betanin—a food colorant with biological activity. Molecular nutrition & food research,

59(1), 36-47.

Estruch, R., Ros, E., Salas-Salvadó, J., Covas, M. I., Corella, D., Arós, F., ... & Lamuela-Raventos, R. M. (2013). Primary prevention of cardiovascular disease with a Mediterranean diet. New England Journal of Medicine, 368(14), 1279-1290.

Fanaei, H., Khayat, S., Kasaeian, A., & Javadimehr, M. (2016). Effect of curcumin on serum brain-derived neurotrophic factor levels in women with premenstrual syndrome: A randomized, double-blind, placebo-controlled trial. Neuropeptides, 56, 25-31.

Faridi, Z., Njike, V. Y., Dutta, S., Ali, A., & Katz, D. L. (2008). Acute dark chocolate and cocoa ingestion and endothelial function: a randomized controlled crossover trial. The American journal of clinical nutrition, 88(1), 58-63.

Farris, W., Mansourian, S., Chang, Y., Lindsley, L., Eckman, E. A., Frosch, M. P., ... & Guénette, S. (2003). Insulin-degrading enzyme regulates the levels of insulin, amyloid β-protein, and the β-amyloid precursor protein intracellular domain in vivo. Proceedings of the National Academy of Sciences, 100(7), 4162-4167.

Farzaei, H. M., Rahimi, R., & Abdollahi, M. (2015). The role of dietary polyphenols in the management of inflammatory bowel disease. Current pharmaceutical biotechnology, 16(3), 196-210.

Fayyaz, S., Aydin, T., Cakir, A., Gasparri, M. L., Benedetti Panici, P., & Ahmad Farooqi, A. (2016). Oleuropein mediated targeting of signaling network in cancer. Current topics in medicinal chemistry, 16(22), 2477-2483

Ferrucci, L., Cherubini, A., Bandinelli, S., Bartali, B., Corsi, A., Lauretani, F., ... & Guralnik, J. M. (2006). Relationship of plasma polyunsaturated fatty acids to circulating inflammatory markers. The Journal of Clinical Endocrinology & Metabolism, 91(2), 439-446.

Fitzpatrick, F. A. (2004). Cyclooxygenase enzymes: regulation and function. Current pharmaceutical design, 10(6), 577-588.

Fleischauer, A. T., & Arab, L. (2001). Garlic and cancer: a critical review of the epidemiologic literature. The Journal of nutrition, 131(3), 1032S-1040S.

Flematti GR, Ghisalberti EL, Dixon KW, Trengove RD (2004) A compound from smoke that promotes seed germination. Science 305, 977.

Flores, G. (2017). Curcuma longa L. extract improves the cortical neural connectivity during the aging process. Neural regeneration research, 12(6), 875.

Folkman, J., & Kalluri, R. (2004). Cancer without disease. Nature, 427(6977), 787-787.

FSANZ (2013). Food Standards Australia and New Zealand, Food Nutrient Database. http://www.foodstandards.gov.au/science/monitoringnutrients/ausnut/foodnutrient/Pages/default.aspx

Forman, H. J., Davies, K. J., & Ursini, F. (2014). How do nutritional antioxidants really work: nucleophilic tone and para-hormesis versus free radical scavenging in vivo. Free Radical Biology and Medicine, 66, 24-35.

Fowsiya, J., & Madhumitha, G. (2017). Preliminary phytochemical analysis, Antioxidant and cytotoxicity test of Carissa edulis Vahl dried fruits. In IOP Conference Series: Materials Science and Engineering (Vol. 263, No. 2, p. 022018). IOP Publishing.

Frei, B., & Higdon, J. V. (2003). Antioxidant activity of tea polyphenols in vivo: evidence from animal studies. The Journal of nutrition, 133(10), 3275S-3284S.

Frondoza, C. G., Sohrabi, A., Polotsky, A., Phan, P. V., Hungerford, D. S., & Lindmark, L. (2004). An in vitro screening assay for inhibitors of proinflammatory mediators in herbal extracts using human synoviocyte cultures. In Vitro Cellular & Developmental Biology-Animal, 40(3), 95-101.

Fujioka, K., Greenway, F., Sheard, J., & Ying, Y. (2006). The effects of grapefruit on weight and insulin resistance: relationship to the metabolic syndrome. Journal of medicinal food, 9(1), 49-54.

Fung J. (2016). The Obesity Code. Unlocking the secrets of weight loss. Scribe, Melbourne.

Fung, J. (2018). The Diabetes Code: Prevent and Reverse Type 2 Diabetes Naturally. Scribe, Melbourne.

Furman R. (2018). Defeating Demntia. What you can do to prevent Alzheimer's and other forms of dementia. Revell, Michigan.

Gadi, D., Bnouham, M., Aziz, M., Ziyyat, A., Legssyer, A., Bruel, A., ... & Mekhfi, H. (2012). Flavonoids purified from parsley inhibit human blood platelet aggregation and adhesion to collagen under flow. Journal of Complementary and Integrative Medicine, 9(1).

Galati, G., & O'brien, P. J. (2004). Potential toxicity of flavonoids and other dietary phenolics: significance for their chemopreventive and anticancer properties. Free Radical Biology and Medicine, 37(3), 287-303.

Galeone, C., Pelucchi, C., Levi, F., Negri, E., Franceschi, S., Talamini, R., ... & La Vecchia, C. (2006). Onion and garlic use and human cancer−. The American journal of clinical nutrition, 84(5), 1027-1032.

Gao, X., Cassidy, A., Schwarzschild, M. A., Rimm, E. B., & Ascherio, A. (2012). Habitual intake of dietary flavonoids and risk of Parkinson disease. Neurology, 78(15), 1138-1145.

Gardener, H., Dong, C., Rundek, T., McLaughlin, C., Cheung, K., Elkind, M., ... & Wright, C. (2017). Diet Clusters in Relation to Cognitive Performance and Decline in the Northern Manhattan Study (S15. 003). Neurology, 88(16 Supplement), S15-003.

Garg, M. L., Blake, R. J., Wills, R. B., & Clayton, E. H. (2007). Macadamia nut consumption modulates favourably risk factors for coronary artery disease in hypercholesterolemic subjects. Lipids, 42(6), 583-587.

Gately, S., & Li, W. W. (2004). Multiple roles of COX-2 in tumor angiogenesis: a target for antiangiogenic therapy. In Seminars in Oncology (Vol. 31, pp. 2-11).

Gee, L. C., & Ahluwalia, A. (2016). Dietary nitrate lowers blood pressure: epidemiological, pre-clinical experimental and clinical trial evidence. Current hypertension reports, 18(2), 17.

Giacosa, A., Morazzoni, P., Bombardelli, E., Riva, A., Bianchi Porro, G., & Rondanelli, M. (2015). Can nausea and vomiting be treated with ginger extract. Eur Rev Med Pharmacol Sci, 19(7), 1291-6.

Gibson-Moore, H., & Spiro, A. (2017). Can turmeric really prevent cancer?. Nutrition Bulletin, 42(2), 141-147.

Gillespie D. (2013). 'Toxic Oil: Why Vegetable Oil Will Kill You & how to Save Yourself'. Viking Publishers.

Gillespie D. (2015). 'Eat real food. The only solution to permanent weight-loss and Disease prevention.' Pan MacMillion Australia.

Giordano, D., Beta, T., Vanara, F., & Blandino, M. (2018). Influence of Agricultural Management on Phytochemicals of Colored Corn Genotypes (Zea mays L.). Part 1: Nitrogen Fertilization. Journal of agricultural and food chemistry, 66(17), 4300-4308.

Goff S. A.,& Klee H. J. (2006). Plant volatile compounds: sensory cues for health and nutritional value?. Science, 311 (5762), 815-819.

Goggins, W. B., & Wong, G. (2009). Cancer among Asian Indians/Pakistanis living in the United States: low incidence and generally above average survival. Cancer Causes & Control, 20(5), 635-643.

González-Castejón, M., & Rodriguez-Casado, A. (2011). Dietary phytochemicals and their potential effects on obesity: a review. Pharmacological Research, 64(5), 438-455.

Grabacka, M. M., Gawin, M., & Pierzchalska, M. (2014). Phytochemical modulators of mitochondria: The search for chemopreventive agents and supportive therapeutics. Pharmaceuticals, 7(9), 913-942.

Grassi, D., Lippi, C., Necozione, S., Desideri, G., & Ferri, C. (2005). Short-term administration of dark chocolate is followed by a significant increase in insulin sensitivity and a decrease in blood pressure in healthy persons. The American journal of clinical nutrition, 81(3), 611-614.

Grassi, D., Necozione, S., Lippi, C., Croce, G., Valeri, L., Pasqualetti, P., ... & Ferri, C. (2005). Cocoa reduces blood pressure and insulin resistance and improves endothelium-dependent vasodilation in hypertensives. Hypertension, 46(2), 398-405.

Grassi, D., Draijer, R., Desideri, G., Mulder, T., & Ferri, C. (2015). Black tea lowers blood pressure and wave reflections in fasted and postprandial conditions in hypertensive patients: a randomised study. Nutrients, 7(2), 1037-1051.

Gray, N. E., Harris, C. J., Quinn, J. F., & Soumyanath, A. (2016). Centella asiatica modulates antioxidant and mitochondrial pathways and improves cognitive function in mice. Journal of ethnopharmacology, 180, 78-86.

Grzanna, R., Lindmark, L., & Frondoza, C. G. (2005). Ginger—an herbal medicinal product with broad anti-inflammatory actions. Journal of medicinal food, 8(2), 125-132.

Grice, I. D., Rogers, K. L., & Griffiths, L. R. (2011). Isolation of bioactive compounds that relate to the anti-platelet activity of Cymbopogon ambiguus. Evidence-Based Complementary and Alternative Medicine, 2011.

Grosso, G., Godos, J., Galvano, F., & Giovannucci, E. L. (2017). Coffee, caffeine, and health outcomes: an umbrella review. Annual Review of Nutrition, 37(1).

Grosso, G., Marventano, S., Yang, J., Micek, A., Pajak, A., Scalfi, L., ... & Kales, S. N. (2017). A comprehensive meta-analysis on evidence of Mediterranean diet and cardiovascular disease: are individual components equal?. Critical reviews in food science and nutrition, 57(15), 3218-3232.

Gu, Q., Dillon, C. F., Eberhardt, M. S., Wright, J. D., & Burt, V. L. (2015). Preventive aspirin and other antiplatelet medication use among US adults aged≥ 40 years: data from the National Health and Nutrition Examination Survey, 2011–2012. Public Health Reports, 130(6), 643-654.

Gul, H. F., Ilhan, N., Ilhan, N., & Ozercan, I. H. (2017). Effect of Pomegranate Extract and Tangeretin on Specific Pathways in the Rat Breast Cancer Model Induced with DMBA. Multidisciplinary Digital Publishing Institute Proceedings, 1(10), 983.

Guo, C., Liu, S., Guo, Y., Yin, Y., Lin, J., Chen, X., & Sun, M. Z. (2014). Comparative function-structural analysis of antiplatelet and antiradical activities of flavonoid phytochemicals. J Anim Plant Sci, 24, 926-935.

Gupta, P., Kim, B., Kim, S. H., & Srivastava, S. K. (2014). Molecular targets of isothiocyanates in cancer: recent advances. Molecular nutrition & food research, 58(8), 1685-1707.

Gupta, P., Wright, S. E., Kim, S. H., & Srivastava, S. K. (2014b). Phenethyl isothiocyanate: A comprehensive review of anti-cancer mechanisms. Biochimica et Biophysica Acta (BBA)-Reviews on Cancer, 1846(2), 405-424.

Gupta, S. C., Patchva, S., & Aggarwal, B. B. (2013). Therapeutic roles of curcumin: lessons learned from clinical trials. The AAPS journal, 15(1), 195-218.

Gupta, V. K., Singh, R., & Sharma, B. (2017). Phytochemicals mediated signalling pathways and their implications in cancer chemotherapy: Challenges and opportunities in phytochemicals based drug development: A review. Biochemical Compounds, 5(1), 2.

Habauzit, V., Verny, M. A., Milenkovic, D., Barber-Chamoux, N., Mazur, A., Dubray, C., & Morand, C. (2015). Flavanones protect from arterial stiffness in postmenopausal women consuming grapefruit juice for 6 mo: a randomized, controlled, crossover trial. The American journal of clinical nutrition, 102(1), 66-74.

Hajiaghaalipour, F., Khalilpourfarshbafi, M., & Arya, A. (2015). Modulation of glucose transporter protein by dietary flavonoids in type 2 diabetes mellitus. International journal of biological sciences, 11(5), 508.

Halliwell B. and Gutteridge J. M. C. (2015) 'Free Radicals in Biology and Medicine'. Oxford University Press.

Halvorsen, S., Andreotti, F., Jurriën, M., Cattaneo, M., Coccheri, S., Marchioli, R., ... & De Caterina, R. (2014). Aspirin therapy in primary cardiovascular disease prevention: a position paper of the European Society of Cardiology working group on thrombosis. Journal of the American College of Cardiology, 64(3), 319-327.

Haque, A. M., Hashimoto, M., Katakura, M., Hara, Y., & Shido, O. (2008). Green tea catechins prevent cognitive deficits caused by $A\beta 1-40$ in rats. The Journal of nutritional biochemistry, 19(9), 619-626.

Hartmann, T. (2007). From waste products to ecochemicals: fifty years research of plant secondary metabolism. Phytochemistry, 68(22), 2831-2846.

Hashmi, M. A., Khan, A., Hanif, M., Farooq, U., & Perveen, S. (2015). Traditional uses, phytochemistry, and pharmacology of Olea europaea (olive). Evidence-Based Complementary and Alternative Medicine, 2015.

Haslam, S., & Hauser, J. (2004). Noosa's Native Plants. Second Edition. Noosa Integrated Catchment Association.

Haytowitz, D. B., & Bhagwat, S. (2010). USDA database for the oxygen radical absorbance capacity (ORAC) of selected foods, Release 2. US Department of Agriculture, 10-48.

He, F. J., Nowson, C. A., & MacGregor, G. A. (2006). Fruit and vegetable consumption and stroke: meta-analysis of cohort studies. The Lancet, 367(9507), 320-326.

He, S., Simpson, B. K., Sun, H., Ngadi, M. O., Ma, Y., & Huang, T. (2018). Phaseolus vulgaris lectins: A systematic review of characteristics and health implications. Critical reviews in food science and nutrition, 58(1), 70-83.

He, Z. H., Gilli, C., Yue, G. G. L., Bik-San Lau, C., Greger, H., Brecker, L., ... & But, P. P. H. (2012). Anti-angiogenic effects and mechanisms of zerumin A from Alpinia caerulea. Food chemistry, 132(1), 201-208.

He, Z. Y., Shi, C. B., Wen, H., Li, F. L., Wang, B. L., & Wang, J. (2011). Upregulation of p53 expression in patients with colorectal cancer by administration of curcumin. Cancer investigation, 29(3), 208-213.

Hegarty, M. P., Hegarty, E. E., & Wills, R. B. H. (2001). Rural industries research and development corporation.

Heldt, H. W., & Piechulla, B. (2011). 8-Photosynthesis implies the consumption of water. Plant Biochemistry (Fourth Edition). Academic Press, San Diego, 211-239.

Hendrie, G. and Noakes, M. (2017). 'Fruit, Vegetables and Diet Score'. CSIRO.

Henig, R. M. (2000). A monk and two peas: the story of Gregor Mendel and the discovery of genetics. Weidenfeld & Nicolson.

Heimler, D., Romani, A., & Ieri, F. (2017). Plant polyphenol content, soil fertilization and agricultural management: a review. European Food Research and Technology, 1-9.

Henkin, R. I., & Gillis, W. T. (1977). Divergent taste responsiveness to fruit of the tree Antidesma bunius. Nature, 265(5594), 536.

Henry, R. J., Rice, N., Waters, D. L., Kasem, S., Ishikawa, R., Hao, Y., ... & Vaughan, D. (2010). Australian Oryza: utility and conservation. Rice, 3(4), 235-241.

Hercberg, S. (2005). The history of β-carotene and cancers: from observational to intervention studies. What lessons can be drawn for future research on polyphenols?. The American journal of clinical nutrition, 81(1), 218S-222S.

Hernández-Aquino, E., Zarco, N., Casas-Grajales, S., Ramos-Tovar, E., Flores-Beltrán, R. E., Arauz, J., ... & Muriel, P. (2017). Naringenin prevents experimental liver fibrosis by blocking TGFβ-Smad3 and JNK-Smad3 pathways. World journal of gastroenterology, 23(24), 4354.

Hernández-Ramírez, R. U., Galván-Portillo, M. V., Ward, M. H., Agudo, A., González, C. A., Oñate-Ocaña, L. F., ... & López-Carrillo, L. (2009). Dietary intake of polyphenols, nitrate and nitrite and gastric cancer risk in Mexico City. International journal of cancer, 125(6), 1424-1430.

Hess, A., Axmann, R., Rech, J., Finzel, S., Heindl, C., Kreitz, S., ... & Straub, R. H. (2011). Blockade of TNF-α rapidly inhibits pain responses in the central nervous system. Proceedings of the National Academy of Sciences, 108(9), 3731-3736.

Higdon, J. & Drake, V. J. (2013). An Evidence-Based Approach to Phytochemicals and Other Dietary Factors. Second Edition. Thieme, New York.

Hjartåker, A., Knudsen, M. D., Tretli, S., & Weiderpass, E. (2015). Consumption of berries, fruits and vegetables and mortality among 10,000 Norwegian men followed for four decades. European journal of nutrition, 54(4), 599-608.

Hodges, R. E., & Minich, D. M. (2015). Modulation of metabolic detoxification pathways using foods and food-derived components: a scientific review with clinical application. Journal of nutrition and metabolism, 2015.

Holford, P. (2010). *Optimum nutrition for the mind*. Hachette UK.

Hord, N. G., Tang, Y., & Bryan, N. S. (2009). Food sources of nitrates and nitrites: the physiologic context for potential health benefits−. The American journal of clinical nutrition, 90(1), 1-10.

Hou, R., Garner, M., Holmes, C., Osmond, C., Teeling, J., Lau, L., & Baldwin, D. S. (2017). Peripheral inflammatory cytokines and immune balance in Generalised Anxiety Disorder: Case-controlled study. Brain, behavior, and immunity, 62, 212-218.

Howatson, G., McHugh, M. P., Hill, J. A., Brouner, J., Jewell, A. P., Van Someren, K. A., ... & Howatson, S. A. (2010). Influence of tart cherry juice on indices of recovery following marathon running. Scandinavian journal of medicine & science in sports, 20(6), 843-852.

HSu T. (2018) Coffee Drinkers Need Cancer Warning, Judge Rules, Giving Sellers the Jitters. The New York Times, 30 March 2018 cited at https://mobile.nytimes.com/2018/03/30/business/coffee-cancer-warning.html

Hsu, Y. L., Chen, C. Y., Lin, I. P., Tsai, E. M., Kuo, P. L., & Hou, M. F. (2012). 4-Shogaol, an active constituent of dietary ginger, inhibits metastasis of MDA-MB-231 human breast adenocarcinoma cells by decreasing the repression of NF-κB/Snail on RKIP. Journal of agricultural and food chemistry, 60(3), 852-861.

Huang, D. (2016). How sulfur binds to gold; Sweet discovery in leafy greens. Chemistry in Australia, (Jun 2016), 18.

Huang, Y., Li, W., Su, Z. Y., & Kong, A. N. T. (2015). The complexity of the Nrf2 pathway: beyond the antioxidant response. The Journal of nutritional biochemistry, 26(12), 1401-1413.

Hung, W. L., Suh, J. H., & Wang, Y. (2017). Chemistry and health effects of furanocoumarins in grapefruit. Journal of food and drug analysis, 25(1), 71-83.

Hungerford, C. (2012). Good Health in the 21st Century: A Family Doctor's Unconventional Guide. Scribe Publications.

Huxley, R., Lee, C. M. Y., Barzi, F., Timmermeister, L., Czernichow, S., Perkovic, V., ... & Woodward, M. (2009). Coffee, decaffeinated coffee, and tea consumption in relation to incident type 2 diabetes mellitus: a systematic review with meta-analysis. Archives of internal medicine, 169(22), 2053-2063.

Hyman, M. (2016). 'Eat fat, get thin: Why the fat we eat is the key to sustained weight loss and vibrant health'. Hachette UK.

Imran, M., Arshad, M. S., Butt, M. S., Kwon, J. H., Arshad, M. U., & Sultan, M. T. (2017). Mangiferin: a natural miracle bioactive compound against lifestyle related disorders. Lipids in health and disease, 16(1), 84.

Ishikawa, H., Saeki, T., Otani, T., Suzuki, T., Shimozuma, K., Nishino, H., ... & Morimoto, K. (2006). Aged garlic extract prevents a decline of NK cell number and activity in patients with advanced cancer. The Journal of nutrition, 136(3), 816S-820S.

Itokawa Y. (1976) Kanehiro Takaki (1849-1920) A Biographical Sketch. Journal of Nutrition 106: 581-588.

Iuvone, T., De Filippis, D., Esposito, G., D'Amico, A., & Izzo, A. A. (2006). The spice sage and its active ingredient rosmarinic acid protect PC12 cells from amyloid-β peptide-induced neurotoxicity. Journal of Pharmacology and Experimental Therapeutics, 317(3), 1143-1149.

Jacka F. (2019). 'Brain Changer. The latest cutting-edge science on how diet can affect your risk of anxiety and depression, and influence the health of your brain.' Pan Macmillan Australia.

Jacka, F. N., O'Neil, A., Opie, R., Itsiopoulos, C., Cotton, S., Mohebbi, M., ... & Brazionis, L. (2017). A randomised controlled trial of dietary improvement for adults with major depression (the 'SMILES'trial). BMC medicine, 15(1), 23.

Jacob, K., Periago, M. J., Böhm, V., & Berruezo, G. R. (2008). Influence of lycopene and vitamin C from tomato juice on biomarkers of oxidative stress and inflammation. British Journal of Nutrition, 99(1), 137-146.

Jaleel, C. A., Manivannan, P., Wahid, A., Farooq, M., Al-Juburi, H. J., Somasundaram, R. A. M. A. M. U. R. T. H. Y., & Panneerselvam, R. (2009). Drought stress in plants: a review on morphological characteristics and pigments composition. Int J Agric Biol, 11(1), 100-105.

Jamieson, N., Sirdaarta, J., & Cock, I. E. (2014). The anti-proliferative properties of Australian plants with high antioxidant capacities against cancer cell lines. Pharmacognosy Communications, 4(4), 71.

Jang, Y., Lee, J. H., Kim, O. Y., Park, H. Y., & Lee, S. Y. (2001). Consumption of whole grain and legume powder reduces insulin demand, lipid peroxidation, and plasma homocysteine concentrations in patients with coronary artery disease: randomized controlled clinical trial. Arteriosclerosis, thrombosis, and vascular biology, 21(12), 2065-2071.

Jansen, M. A. (2002). Ultraviolet-B radiation effects on plants: induction of morphogenic responses. Physiologia Plantarum, 116(3), 423-429.

Jarvill-Taylor, K. J., Anderson, R. A., & Graves, D. J. (2001). A hydroxychalcone derived from cinnamon functions as a mimetic for insulin in 3T3-L1 adipocytes. Journal of the American College of Nutrition, 20(4), 327-336.

Jeandet, P., Hébrard, C., Deville, M. A., Cordelier, S., Dorey, S., Aziz, A., & Crouzet, J. (2014). Deciphering the role of phytoalexins in plant-microorganism interactions and human health. Molecules, 19(11), 18033-18056.

Jeffreys, D. (2008).'Aspirin: the remarkable story of a wonder drug.' Bloomsbury Publishing USA.

Jeong, C. H., Bode, A. M., Pugliese, A., Cho, Y. Y., Kim, H. G., Shim, J. H., ... & Dong, Z. (2009). [6]-Gingerol suppresses colon cancer growth by targeting leukotriene A4 hydrolase. Cancer research, 69(13), 5584-5591.

Jensen, M. K., Koh-Banerjee, P., Franz, M., Sampson, L., Grønbæk, M., & Rimm, E. B. (2006). Whole grains, bran, and germ in relation to homocysteine and markers of glycemic control, lipids, and inflammation−. The American journal of clinical nutrition, 83(2), 275-283.

Jiang, J. Z., Ye, J., Jin, G. Y., Piao, H. M., Cui, H., Zheng, M. Y., ... & Yan, G. H. (2017). Asiaticoside Mitigates the Allergic Inflammation by Abrogating the Degranulation of Mast Cells. Journal of agricultural and food chemistry, 65(37), 8128-8135.

Jochmann, N., Lorenz, M., von Krosigk, A., Martus, P., Böhm, V., Baumann, G., ... & Stangl, V. (2008). The efficacy of black tea in ameliorating endothelial function is equivalent to that of green tea. British Journal of Nutrition, 99(4), 863-868.

Johnson, J. J. (2011). Carnosol: a promising anti-cancer and anti-inflammatory agent. Cancer letters, 305(1), 1-7.

Jorjong, S., Butkhup, L., & Samappito, S. (2015). Phytochemicals and antioxidant capacities of Mao-Luang (Antidesma bunius L.) cultivars from Northeastern Thailand. Food chemistry, 181, 248-255.

Josling, P. (2001). Preventing the common cold with a garlic supplement: a double-blind, placebo-controlled survey. Advances in therapy, 18(4), 189-193.

Jung, H. Y., Lee, D., Ryu, H. G., Choi, B. H., Go, Y., Lee, N., ... & Yoon, J. H. (2017). Myricetin improves endurance capacity and mitochondrial density by activating SIRT1 and PGC-1α. Scientific Reports, 7.

Justesen, U., Knuthsen, P., & Leth, T. (1998). Quantitative analysis of flavonols, flavones, and flavanones in fruits, vegetables and beverages by high-performance liquid chromatography with photo-diode array and mass spectrometric detection. Journal of Chromatography A, 799(1), 101-110.

Kappelmann, N., Lewis, G., Dantzer, R., Jones, P. B., & Khandaker, G. M. (2016). Antidepressant activity of anti-cytokine treatment: a systematic review and meta-analysis of clinical trials of chronic inflammatory conditions. Molecular psychiatry. October.

Katsukawa, M., Nakata, R., Takizawa, Y., Hori, K., Takahashi, S., & Inoue, H. (2010). Citral, a component of lemongrass oil, activates PPARα and γ and suppresses COX-2 expression. Biochimica et Biophysica Acta (BBA)-Molecular and Cell Biology of Lipids, 1801(11), 1214-1220.

Kennedy, D. O. (2014). 'Plants and the human brain.' Oxford University Press.

Kennedy, D. O., Pace, S., Haskell, C., Okello, E. J., Milne, A., & Scholey, A. B. (2006). Effects of cholinesterase inhibiting sage (Salvia officinalis) on mood, anxiety and performance on a psychological stressor battery. Neuropsychopharmacology, 31(4), 845-852.

Kensler, T. W., Ng, D., Carmella, S. G., Chen, M., Jacobson, L. P., Muñoz, A., ... & Fahey, J. W. (2011). Modulation of the metabolism of airborne pollutants by glucoraphanin-rich and sulforaphane-rich broccoli sprout beverages in Qidong, China. Carcinogenesis, 33(1), 101-107.

Khalid, S., Barfoot, K. L., May, G., Lamport, D. J., Reynolds, S. A., & Williams, C. M. (2017). Effects of acute blueberry flavonoids on mood in children and young adults. Nutrients, 9(2), 158.

Khan, A., Safdar, M., Khan, M. M. A., Khattak, K. N., & Anderson, R. A. (2003). Cinnamon improves glucose and lipids of people with type 2 diabetes. Diabetes care, 26(12), 3215-3218.

Khan, N. A., Walk, A. M., Edwards, C. G., Jones, A. R., Cannavale, C. N., Thompson, S. V., ... & Holscher, H. D. (2018). Macular Xanthophylls Are Related to Intellectual Ability among Adults with Overweight and Obesity. Nutrients, 10(4), 396.

Kim, H., Youn, K., Yun, E. Y., Hwang, J. S., Jeong, W. S., Ho, C. T., & Jun, M. (2015). Oleic acid ameliorates Aβ-induced inflammation by downregulation of COX-2 and iNOS via NFκB signaling pathway. Journal of Functional Foods, 14, 1-11.

Kim, H. G., Ju, M. S., Shim, J. S., Kim, M. C., Lee, S. H., Huh, Y., ... & Oh, M. S. (2010). Mulberry fruit protects dopaminergic neurons in toxin-induced Parkinson's disease models. British Journal of Nutrition, 104(1), 8-16.

Kim, M. K., Suh, D. H., Kim, B., & Song, Y. S. (2014). Cellular stress responses and cancer: new mechanistic insights on anticancer effect by phytochemicals. Phytochemistry reviews, 13(1), 207-221.

Kim, Y., Narayanan, S., & Chang, K. O. (2010). Inhibition of influenza virus replication by plant-derived isoquercetin. Antiviral research, 88(2), 227-235.

Kleemann, R., Verschuren, L., Morrison, M., Zadelaar, S., van Erk, M. J., Wielinga, P. Y., & Kooistra, T. (2011). Anti-inflammatory, anti-proliferative and anti-atherosclerotic effects of quercetin in human in vitro and in vivo models. Atherosclerosis, 218(1), 44-52.

Ko, E. Y., Cho, S. H., Kang, K., Kim, G., Lee, J. H., Jeon, Y. J., ... & Kim, K. N. (2017). Anti-inflammatory activity of hydrosols from Tetragonia tetragonoides in LPS-induced RAW 264.7 cells. EXCLI journal, 16, 521.

Kuptniratsaikul, V., Dajpratham, P., Taechaarpornkul, W., Buntragulpoontawee, M., Lukkanapichonchut, P., Chootip, C., ... & Laongpech, S. (2014). Efficacy and safety of Curcuma domestica extracts compared with ibuprofen in patients with knee osteoarthritis: a multicenter study. Clinical interventions in aging, 9, 451.

Konczak, I. (2015). Health attributes of Indigenous Australian Plants. Chapter 9. In: Cherikoff V. (Ed). Wild Foods. Looking back 60,years for clues to our future survival. New Holland Publishers, London.

Konczak, I., Zabaras, D., Dunstan, M., Aguas, P., Roulfe, P., & Pavan, A. (2009). Health benefits of Australian native foods: an evaluation of health-enhancing compounds. Australia: Rural Industries Research and Development Corporation, Publication 09/133.

Konczak, I., Zabaras, D., Dunstan, M., & Aguas, P. (2010). Antioxidant capacity and hydrophilic phytochemicals in commercially grown native Australian fruits. Food Chemistry, 123(4), 1048-1054.

Konczak, I., Sakulnarmrat, K. and Bull, M. (2012) Potential Physiological Activities of Selected Australian Herbs and Fruits. Publication No. 11/097. Rural Industries Research and Development Corporation. Barton, ACT, Australia.

Korat, A. V. A., Willett, W. C., & Hu, F. B. (2014). Diet, lifestyle, and genetic risk factors for type 2 diabetes: a review from the Nurses' Health Study, Nurses' Health Study 2, and Health Professionals' Follow-up Study. Current nutrition reports, 3(4), 345-354.

Krikorian R., Shidler M. D., Nash T. A., Kalt W., Vinqvist-Tymchuk M. R., Shukitt-Hale B. and Joseph J. A. (2010). Blueberry supplementation improves memory in older adults. Journal of Agricultural and Food Chemistry 58:3996 – 4000.

Kummerow, F. A. (2014). Two lipids in the diet, rather than cholesterol, are responsible for heart failure and stroke. Clinical Lipidology, 9(2), 189-204.

Kuo, P. L., Hsu, Y. L., Huang, M. S., Tsai, M. J., & Ko, Y. C. (2011). Ginger suppresses phthalate ester-induced airway remodeling. Journal of agricultural and food chemistry, 59(7), 3429-3438.

Kuptniratsaikul, V., Thanakhumtorn, S., Chinswangwatanakul, P., Wattanamongkonsil, L., & Thamlikitkul, V. (2009). Efficacy and safety of Curcuma domestica extracts in patients with knee osteoarthritis. The Journal of Alternative and Complementary Medicine, 15(8), 891-897.

Kuriyama, S., Shimazu, T., Ohmori, K., Kikuchi, N., Nakaya, N., Nishino, Y., ... & Tsuji, I. (2006). Green tea consumption and mortality due to cardiovascular disease, cancer, and all causes in Japan: the Ohsaki study. Jama, 296(10), 1255-1265.

Labban, L. (2014). Medicinal and pharmacological properties of Turmeric (Curcuma longa): A review. Journal of Pharmaceutical and Biomedical Sciences, 5(1), 17-23.

Labrecque, L., Lamy, S., Chapus, A., Mihoubi, S., Durocher, Y., Cass, B., ... & Béliveau, R. (2005). Combined inhibition of PDGF and VEGF receptors by ellagic acid, a dietary-derived phenolic compound. Carcinogenesis, 26(4), 821-826.

Lafont, R., & Dinan, L. (2003). Practical uses for ecdysteroids in mammals including humans: and update. Journal of Insect Science, 3 (7), 1-30.

Lagrange, H., Jay-Allgmand, C., & Lapeyrie, F. (2001). Rutin, the phenolglycoside from eucalyptus root exudates, stimulates Pisolithus hyphal growth at picomolar concentrations. New Phytologist, 149(2), 349-355.

Lai, W. K. C., & Kan, M. Y. (2015). Homocysteine-induced endothelial dysfunction. Annals of Nutrition and Metabolism, 67(1), 1-12.

Lakhan, S. E., Ford, C. T., & Tepper, D. (2015). Zingiberaceae extracts for pain: a systematic review and meta-analysis. Nutrition journal, 14(1), 50.

Lakhanpal, P., & Rai, D. K. (2007). Quercetin: a versatile flavonoid. Internet Journal of Medical Update, 2(2), 22-37.

Lako, J., Trenerry, V. C., Wahlqvist, M., Wattanapenpaiboon, N., Sotheeswaran, S., & Premier, R. (2007). Phytochemical flavonols, carotenoids and the antioxidant properties of a wide selection of Fijian fruit, vegetables and other readily available foods. Food Chemistry, 101(4), 1727-1741.

Latz, P. K. (1995). 'Bushfires and Bushtucker.' IAD Press, Alice Springs.

Lee, E. A., Angka, L., Rota, S. G., Hanlon, T., Mitchell, A., Hurren, R., ... & Minden, M. (2015). Targeting mitochondria with avocatin B induces selective leukemia cell death. Cancer research, 75(12), 2478-2488.

Lee, M. S., Wahlqvist, M. L., Chou, Y. C., Fang, W. H., Lee, J. T., Kuan, J. C., ... & Andrews, Z. B. (2014). Turmeric improves post-prandial working memory in pre-diabetes independent of insulin. Asia Pacific journal of clinical nutrition, 23(4), 581.

Leiherer, A., Mündlein, A., & Drexel, H. (2013). Phytochemicals and their impact on adipose tissue inflammation and diabetes. Vascular pharmacology, 58(1), 3-20.

Leiss, K. A., Maltese, F., Choi, Y. H., Verpoorte, R., & Klinkhamer, P. G. (2009). Identification of chlorogenic acid as a resistance factor for thrips in chrysanthemum. Plant Physiology, 150(3), 1567-1575.

Leong, P. K., & Ko, K. M. (2016). Induction of the Glutathione Antioxidant Response/Glutathione Redox Cycling by Nutraceuticals: Mechanism of Protection against Oxidant-induced Cell Death. Current Trends in Nutraceuticals.

Lete, I., & Allué, J. (2016). The effectiveness of ginger in the prevention of nausea and vomiting during pregnancy and chemotherapy. Integrative medicine insights, 11, IMI-S36273.

Lewis, D. A., Fields, W. N., & Shaw, G. P. (1999). A natural flavonoid present in unripe plantain banana pulp (Musa sapientum L. var. paradisiaca) protects the gastric mucosa from aspirin-induced erosions. Journal of ethnopharmacology, 65(3), 283-288.

Li, J. J., & Fang, C. H. (2004). C-reactive protein is not only an inflammatory marker but also a direct cause of cardiovascular diseases. Medical hypotheses, 62(4), 499-506.

Li, N., Jia, X., Chen, C. Y. O., Blumberg, J. B., Song, Y., Zhang, W., ... & Chen, J. (2007). Almond consumption reduces oxidative DNA damage and lipid peroxidation in male smokers. The Journal of nutrition, 137(12), 2717-2722.

Li, Y. R., Li, S., & Lin, C. C. (2018). Effect of resveratrol and pterostilbene on aging and longevity. Biofactors, 44(1), 69-82.

Li, W., Guo, Y., Zhang, C., Wu, R., Yang, A. Y., Gaspar, J., & Kong, A. N. T. (2016). Dietary phytochemicals and cancer chemoprevention: a perspective on oxidative stress, inflammation, and epigenetics. Chemical research in toxicology, 29(12), 2071-2095.

Liao, L. H., Wu, W. Y., & Berenbaum, M. R. (2017). Impacts of dietary phytochemicals in the presence and absence of pesticides on longevity of honey bees (Apis mellifera). Insects, 8(1), 22.

Libby, P. (2006). Inflammation and cardiovascular disease mechanisms–. The American journal of clinical nutrition, 83(2), 456S-460S.

Lieberman, S., & Bruning, N. (2007). Real vitamin & mineral book. Fourth Edition. Avery Pub. Group.

Lien, H. C., Sun, W. M., Chen, Y. H., Kim, H., Hasler, W., & Owyang, C. (2003). Effects of ginger on motion sickness and gastric slow-wave dysrhythmias induced by circular vection. American Journal of Physiology-Gastrointestinal and Liver Physiology, 284(3), G481-G489.

Lihn, A. S., Pedersen, S. B., & Richelsen, B. (2005). Adiponectin: action, regulation and association to insulin sensitivity. Obesity reviews, 6(1), 13-21.

Lim, J. W., Kim, H., & Kim, K. H. (2001). Nuclear factor-[kappa] B regulates cyclooxygenase-2 expression and cell proliferation in human gastric cancer cells. Laboratory Investigation, 81(3), 349.

Lim, S., Moon, M., Oh, H., Kim, H. G., Kim, S. Y., & Oh, M. S. (2014). Ginger improves cognitive function via NGF-induced ERK/CREB activation in the hippocampus of the mouse. The Journal of nutritional biochemistry, 25(10), 1058-1065.

Lim, T. K. (2012a). Edible medicinal and non-medicinal plants (Vol. 1, pp. 656-687). Springer, New York, USA.

Lim, T. K. (2012b). Edible Medicinal And Non-Medicinal Plants: Volume 2, Fruits. Springer, New York, USA.

Lim, T. K. (2012c). Edible Medicinal And Non-Medicinal Plants: Volume 3, Fruits. Springer, New York, USA.

Lim, T. K. (2012d). Edible Medicinal And Non-Medicinal Plants: Volume 4, Fruits. Springer, New York, USA.

Lim, T. K. (2013a). Edible Medicinal And Non-Medicinal Plants: Volume 5, Fruits. Springer, New York, USA.

Lim, T. K. (2013b). Edible Medicinal And Non-Medicinal Plants: Volume 6, Fruits. Springer, New York, USA.

Lim, T. K. (2015). Edible Medicinal And Non-Medicinal Plants: Volume 9, Modifed stems, roots, bulbs. Springer, New York, USA.

Lim, S., Choi, J. G., Moon, M., Kim, H. G., Lee, W., Bak, H. R., ... & Oh, M. S. (2016). An Optimized Combination of Ginger and Peony Root Effectively Inhibits Amyloid-β Accumulation and Amyloid-β-Mediated Pathology in AβPP/PS1 Double-Transgenic Mice. Journal of Alzheimer's Disease, 50(1), 189-200.

Lim, J. Y., Park, C. K., & Hwang, S. W. (2015). Biological roles of resolvins and related substances in the resolution of pain. BioMed research international 2015.

Lin, S. (2018). The Dental Diet: The Surprising Link Between Your Teeth, Real Food, and Life-changing Natural Health. Hay House, Inc.

Lingua, G., Bona, E., Manassero, P., Marsano, F., Todeschini, V., Cantamessa, S., ... & Berta, G. (2013). Arbuscular mycorrhizal fungi and plant growth-promoting pseudomonads increases anthocyanin concentration in strawberry fruits (Fragaria x ananassa var. Selva) in conditions of reduced fertilization. International journal of molecular sciences, 14(8), 16207-16225.

Linnewiel-Hermoni, K., Khanin, M., Danilenko, M., Zango, G., Amosi, Y., Levy, J., & Sharoni, Y. (2015). The anti-cancer effects of carotenoids and other phytonutrients resides in their combined activity. Archives of biochemistry and biophysics, 572, 28-35.

Liu, G., Mi, X. N., Zheng, X. X., Xu, Y. L., Lu, J., & Huang, X. H. (2014). Effects of tea intake on blood pressure: a meta-analysis of randomised controlled trials. British Journal of Nutrition, 112(7), 1043-1054.

Liu, L., Howe, P., Zhou, Y. F., Xu, Z. Q., Hocart, C., & Zhang, R. (2000). Fatty acids and β-carotene in Australian purslane (Portulaca oleracea) varieties. Journal of chromatography A, 893(1), 207-213.

Liu, L. K., Lee, H. J., Shih, Y. W., Chyau, C. C., & Wang, C. J. (2008). Mulberry anthocyanin extracts inhibit LDL oxidation and macrophage-derived foam cell formation induced by oxidative LDL. Journal of food science, 73(6).

Liu, R. H. (2003). Health benefits of fruit and vegetables are from additive and synergistic combinations of phytochemicals. The American journal of clinical nutrition, 78(3), 517S-520S.

Liu, R., Wang, T., Zhang, B., Qin, L., Wu, C., Li, Q., & Ma, L. (2015). Lutein and zeaxanthin supplementation and association with visual function in age-related macular degeneration. Investigative ophthalmology & visual science, 56(1), 252-258.

Lobo, V., Patil, A., Phatak, A., & Chandra, N. (2010). Free radicals, antioxidants and functional foods: Impact on human health. Pharmacognosy reviews, 4(8), 118.

Lotito, S. B., & Frei, B. (2006). Consumption of flavonoid-rich foods and increased plasma antioxidant capacity in humans: cause, consequence, or epiphenomenon?. Free Radical Biology and Medicine, 41(12), 1727-1746.

Lopez, M. S., Dempsey, R. J., & Vemuganti, R. (2015). Resveratrol neuroprotection in stroke and traumatic CNS injury. Neurochemistry international, 89, 75-82.

Lopresti, A. L. (2017). Salvia (sage): a review of its potential cognitive-enhancing and protective effects. Drugs in R&D, 17(1), 53-64.

Llorach, R., Martínez-Sánchez, A., Tomás-Barberán, F. A., Gil, M. I., & Ferreres, F. (2008). Characterisation of polyphenols and antioxidant properties of five lettuce varieties and escarole. Food chemistry, 108(3), 1028-1038.

Ludy, M. J., Moore, G. E., & Mattes, R. D. (2011). The effects of capsaicin and capsiate on energy balance: critical review and meta-analyses of studies in humans. Chemical senses, 37(2), 103-121.

Luo, Y., & Wang, Q. (2012). Bioactive compounds in corn. Cereals and Pulses: Nutraceutical properties and health benefits, 85-103.

Lyle, S. (2011). *Eat Smart Stay Well*. David Bateman Publishing Auckland, distributed by CSIRO Publishing, Collingwood.

Ma, L., & Lin, X. M. (2010). Effects of lutein and zeaxanthin on aspects of eye health. Journal of the Science of Food and Agriculture, 90(1), 2-12.

Ma, L., Yan, S. F., Huang, Y. M., Lu, X. R., Qian, F., Pang, H. L., ... & Wang, X. (2012). Effect of lutein and zeaxanthin on macular pigment and visual function in patients with early age-related macular degeneration. Ophthalmology, 119(11), 2290-2297.

Madhu, K., Chanda, K., & Saji, M. J. (2013). Safety and efficacy of Curcuma longa extract in the treatment of painful knee osteoarthritis: a randomized placebo-controlled trial. Inflammopharmacology, 21(2), 129-136.

Madonna, R., & De Caterina, R. (2009). Prolonged exposure to high insulin impairs the endothelial PI3-kinase/Akt/nitric oxide signalling. Thrombosis and haemostasis, 101(02), 345-350.

Magee, E. (2008). 'Food Synergy: Unleash Hundreds of Powerful Healing Food Combinations to Fight Disease and Live Well.' Rodale.

Maki, K. C., Reeves, M. S., Farmer, M., Yasunaga, K., Matsuo, N., Katsuragi, Y., ... & Blumberg, J. B. (2009). Green tea catechin consumption enhances exercise-induced abdominal fat loss in overweight and obese adults. The Journal of nutrition, 139(2), 264-270.

Mallikarjuna, N., Kranthi, K. R., Jadhav, D. R., Kranthi, S., & Chandra, S. (2004). Influence of foliar chemical compounds on the development of Spodoptera litura (Fab.) in interspecific derivatives of groundnut. Journal of Applied Entomology, 128(5), 321-328.

Martin, C., Zhang, Y., Tonelli, C., & Petroni, K. (2013). Plants, diet, and health. Annual review of plant biology, 64, 19-46.

Masibo, M., & He, Q. (2008). Major mango polyphenols and their potential significance to human health. Comprehensive Reviews in Food Science and Food Safety, 7(4), 309-319.

Mashhadi, N. S., Ghiasvand, R., Askari, G., Hariri, M., Darvishi, L., & Mofid, M. R. (2013). Anti-oxidative and anti-inflammatory effects of ginger in health and physical activity: review of current evidence. International journal of preventive medicine, 4(Suppl 1), S36.

Matsumoto, S., Nakanishi, R., Li, D., Alani, A., Rezaeian, P., Prabhu, S., ... & Hamal, S. (2016). Aged Garlic Extract Reduces Low Attenuation Plaque in Coronary Arteries of Patients with Metabolic Syndrome in a Prospective Randomized Double-Blind Study–3. The Journal of nutrition, 146(2), 427S-432S.

McCullough, M. L., Chevaux, K., Jackson, L., Preston, M., Martinez, G., Schmitz, H. H., ... & Hollenberg, N. K. (2006). Hypertension, the Kuna, and the epidemiology of flavanols. Journal of cardiovascular pharmacology, 47, S103-S109.

McCrea, C. E., West, S. G., Kris-Etherton, P. M., Lambert, J. D., Gaugler, T. L., Teeter, D. L., ... & Skulas-Ray, A. C. (2015). Effects of culinary spices and psychological stress on postprandial lipemia and lipase activity: results of a randomized crossover study and in vitro experiments. Journal of translational medicine, 13(1), 7.

McDougall, G. J., Shpiro, F., Dobson, P., Smith, P., Blake, A., & Stewart, D. (2005). Different polyphenolic components of soft fruits inhibit α-amylase and α-glucosidase. Journal of agricultural and food chemistry, 53(7), 2760-2766.

McGuire M. (2016). Your Food. Where your food comes from and how it is produced. Custom Publishing, Strawberry Hills NSW.

McFarlane A. (2010). 'Organic Vegetable Gardening.' HarperCollins Publishers, Sydney.

McFarlane A. (2011). 'Organic Fruit Growing.' HarperCollins Publishers, Sydney.

McKenzie, R. (2012). Australia's poisonous plants, fungi and cyanobacteria: a guide to species of medical and veterinary importance. CSIRO.

McNeil, J. J., Woods, R. L., Nelson, M. R., Reid, C. M., ... and A.M. Murray, for the ASPREE Investigator Group (2018) Effect of Aspirin on Disability-free Survival in the Healthy Elderly. The New England Journal of Medicine DOI: 10.1056/NEJMoa1800722.

Meghwal, M., & Goswami, T. K. (2013). Piper nigrum and piperine: an update. Phytotherapy Research, 27(8), 1121-1130.

Menendez, J. A., Joven, J., Aragonès, G., Barrajón-Catalán, E., Beltrán-Debón, R., Borrás-Linares, I., ... & Garcia-Heredia, A. (2013). Xenohormetic and anti-aging activity of secoiridoid polyphenols present in extra virgin olive oil: a new family of gerosuppressant agents. Cell Cycle, 12(4), 555-578.

Menendez, J. A., Vellon, L., Colomer, R., & Lupu, R. (2005). Oleic acid, the main mono-unsaturated fatty acid of olive oil, suppresses her-2/neu (erb b-2) expression and synergistically enhances the growth inhibitory effects of trastuzumab (herceptin™) in breast cancer cells with her-2/neu oncogene amplification. Annals of oncology, 16(3), 359-371.

Mercola, J. (2017). 'Fat for Fuel: A Revolutionary Diet to Combat Cancer, Boost Brain Power, and Increase Your Energy.' Hay House, Inc.

Mertens-Talcott, S. U., Jilma-Stohlawetz, P., Rios, J., Hingorani, L., & Derendorf, H. (2006). Absorption, metabolism, and antioxidant effects of pomegranate (Punica granatum L.) polyphenols after ingestion of a standardized extract in healthy human volunteers. Journal of agricultural and food chemistry, 54(23), 8956-8961.

Miller, D. M., Singh, I. N., Wang, J. A., & Hall, E. D. (2015). Nrf2–ARE activator carnosic acid decreases mitochondrial dysfunction, oxidative damage and neuronal cytoskeletal degradation following traumatic brain injury in mice. Experimental neurology, 264, 103-110.

Miller, J. A., Hakim, I. A., Chew, W., Thompson, P., Thomson, C. A., & Chow, H. S. (2010). Adipose tissue accumulation of d-limonene with the consumption of a lemonade preparation rich in d-limonene content. Nutrition and cancer, 62(6), 783-788.

Miller, J. A., Thompson, P. A., Hakim, I. A., Chow, H. H. S., & Thomson, C. A. (2011). d-Limonene: a bioactive food component from citrus and evidence for a potential role in breast cancer prevention and treatment. Oncology Reviews, 5(1), 31-42.

Miller, J. A., Lang, J. E., Ley, M., Nagle, R., Hsu, C. H., Thompson, P. A., ... & Chow, H. S. (2013). Human breast tissue disposition and bioactivity of limonene in women with early-stage breast cancer. Cancer Prevention Research, 6(6), 577-584.

Min, K., Freeman, C., Kang, H., & Choi, S. U. (2015). The regulation by phenolic compounds of soil organic matter dynamics under a changing environment. BioMed research international, 2015.

Minger D. (2013). 'Death by Food Pyramid. How shoddy science, sketchy politics and shady special interests ruined your health ... and how to reclaim it.' Primal Blueprint Publishing, Malibu, California.

Mitchell, A. E., Hong, Y. J., Koh, E., Barrett, D. M., Bryant, D. E., Denison, R. F., & Kaffka, S. (2007). Ten-year comparison of the influence of organic and conventional crop management practices on the content of flavonoids in tomatoes. Journal of Agricultural and Food Chemistry, 55(15), 6154-6159.

Mizrahi, A., Knekt, P., Montonen, J., Laaksonen, M. A., Heliövaara, M., & Järvinen, R. (2009). Plant foods and the risk of cerebrovascular diseases: a potential protection of fruit consumption. British journal of nutrition, 102(7), 1075-1083.

Moeller, S. M., Voland, R., Tinker, L., Blodi, B. A., Klein, M. L., Gehrs, K. M., ... & Parekh, N. (2008). Associations between age-related nuclear cataract and lutein and zeaxanthin in the diet and serum in the carotenoids in the age-related eye disease study (CAREDS), an ancillary study of the Women's Health Initiative. Archives of ophthalmology, 126(3), 354-364.

Mohanty, S., & Cock, I. E. (2012). The chemotherapeutic potential of Terminalia ferdinandiana: Phytochemistry and bioactivity. Pharmacognosy reviews, 6(11), 29.

Møller, P. (2013). Gastrophysics in the brain and body. Flavour, 2(1), 8.

Montes de Oca, M. K., Pearlman, R. L., McClees, S. F., Strickland, R., & Afaq, F. (2017). Phytochemicals for the Prevention of Photocarcinogenesis. Photochemistry and photobiology, 93(4), 956-974.

Monti, S. M., Ritieni, A., Sacchi, R., Skog, K., Borgen, E., & Fogliano, V. (2001). Characterization of phenolic compounds in virgin olive oil and their effect on the formation of carcinogenic/mutagenic heterocyclic amines in a model system. Journal of agricultural and food chemistry, 49(8), 3969-3975.

Morgan, M. J., & Liu, Z. G. (2011). Crosstalk of reactive oxygen species and NF-κB signaling. Cell research, 21(1), 103.

Morowitz, M. J., Carlisle, E. M., & Alverdy, J. C. (2011). Contributions of intestinal bacteria to nutrition and metabolism in the critically ill. Surgical Clinics, 91(4), 771-785.

Morris, M. C., Evans, D. A., Tangney, C. C., Bienias, J. L., & Wilson, R. S. (2006). Associations of vegetable and fruit consumption with age-related cognitive change. Neurology, 67(8), 1370-1376.

Morris, M. C. (2018). Diet for the Mind: The Latest Science on What to Eat to Prevent Alzheimer's and Cognitive Decline. Pan Macmillan.

Moskaug, J. Ø., Carlsen, H., Myhrstad, M. C., & Blomhoff, R. (2005). Polyphenols and glutathione synthesis regulation. The American Journal of Clinical Nutrition, 81(1), 277S-283S.

Mucci, L. A., & Wilson, K. M. (2008). Acrylamide intake through diet and human cancer risk. Journal of agricultural and food chemistry, 56(15), 6013-6019.

Müller, V., Lankes, C., Zimmermann, B. F., Noga, G., & Hunsche, M. (2013). Centelloside accumulation in leaves of Centella asiatica is determined by resource partitioning between primary and secondary metabolism while influenced by supply levels of either nitrogen, phosphorus or potassium. Journal of plant physiology, 170(13), 1165-1175.

Munro, I. A., & Garg, M. L. (2008). 15 Nutrient Composition and Health Beneficial Effects of Macadamia Nuts. Tree nuts: Composition, phytochemicals, and health effects, 249.

Mursu, J., Voutilainen, S., Nurmi, T., Rissanen, T. H., Virtanen, J. K., Kaikkonen, J., ... & Salonen, J. T. (2004). Dark chocolate consumption increases HDL cholesterol concentration and chocolate fatty acids may inhibit lipid peroxidation in healthy humans. Free Radical Biology and Medicine, 37(9), 1351-1359.

Murugaiyah, V., & Mattson, M. P. (2015). Neurohormetic phytochemicals: An evolutionary−bioenergetic perspective. Neurochemistry international, 89, 271-280.

Nagao, M., Honda, M., Seino, Y., Yahagi, T., & Sugimura, T. (1977). Mutagenicities of smoke condensates and the charred surface of fish and meat. Cancer Letters, 2(4), 221-226.

Nagata, N., Xu, L., Kohno, S., Ushida, Y., Aoki, Y., Umeda, R., ... & Takahashi, C. (2017). Glucoraphanin ameliorates obesity and insulin resistance through adipose tissue browning and reduction of metabolic endotoxemia in mice. Diabetes, 66(5), 1222-1236.

Nakachi, K., Suemasu, K., Suga, K., Takeo, T., Imai, K., & Higashi, Y. (1998). Influence of drinking green tea on breast cancer malignancy among Japanese patients. Cancer Science, 89(3), 254-261.

Napier K. M. (1998). 'Eat to Heal. The phytochemica diet and nutrition plan.' Warner Books Inc, New York.

Nareika, A., Im, Y. B., Game, B. A., Slate, E. I I., Sanders, J. J., London, S. D., ... & Huang, Y. (2008). High glucose enhances lipopolysaccharide-stimulated CD14 expression in U937 mononuclear cells by increasing nuclear factor κB and AP-1 activities. Journal of Endocrinology, 196(1), 45-55.

Navarrete, S., Alarcón, M., & Palomo, I. (2015). Aqueous extract of tomato (Solanum lycopersicum L.) and ferulic acid reduce the expression of TNF-α and IL-1β in LPS-activated macrophages. Molecules, 20(8), 15319-15329.

Navarro, S. L., Li, F., & Lampe, J. W. (2011). Mechanisms of action of isothiocyanates in cancer chemoprevention: an update. Food & function, 2(10), 579-587.

Netzel, M., Netzel, G., Tian, Q., Schwartz, S., & Konczak, I. (2007). Native Australian fruits—a novel source of antioxidants for food. Innovative food science & emerging technologies, 8(3), 339-346.

Nielsen, S. E., Young, J. F., Daneshvar, B., Lauridsen, S. T., Knuthsen, P., Sandström, B., & Dragsted, L. O. (1999). Effect of parsley (Petroselinum crispum) intake on urinary apigenin excretion, blood antioxidant enzymes and biomarkers for oxidative stress in human subjects. British Journal of Nutrition, 81(6), 447-455.

DiNicolantonio J. and Fung J. (2019). 'The Longevity Solution. Rediscovering Centuries-Old Secrets to a Healthy, Long Life.' Victory Belt Publishing, Las Vegas.

Nitteranon, V., Zhang, G., Darien, B. J., & Parkin, K. (2011). Isolation and synergism of in vitro anti-inflammatory and quinone reductase (QR) inducing agents from the fruits of Morinda citrifolia (noni). Food research international, 44(7), 2271-2277.

Noratto, G., Carrion-Rabanal, R., Medina, G., Mencia, A., Mohanty, I., Gonzalez, D., & Murphy, K. (2015). Quinoa protective effects against obesity-induced intestinal inflammation. The FASEB Journal, 29(1_supplement), 602-9.

O'Dea, K. (1984). Marked improvement in carbohydrate and lipid metabolism in diabetic Australian Aborigines after temporary reversion to traditional lifestyle. Diabetes, 33(6), 596-603.

O'Kennedy, N., Crosbie, L., Whelan, S., Luther, V., Horgan, G., Broom, J. I., ... & Duttaroy, A. K. (2006). Effects of tomato extract on platelet function: a double-blinded crossover study in healthy humans–. The American journal of clinical nutrition, 84(3), 561-569.

Ong, W. Y., Farooqui, T., Ho, C. F. Y., Ng, Y. K., & Farooqui, A. A. (2017). Use of Phytochemicals against Neuroinflammation. Neuroprotective Effects of Phytochemicals in Neurological Disorders, 1.

Orhan, I. E. (2012). Centella asiatica (L.) Urban: from traditional medicine to modern medicine with neuroprotective potential. Evidence-based complementary and alternative medicine, 2012.

Ormsbee, M. J., Lox, J., & Arciero, P. J. (2013). Beetroot juice and exercise performance. Nutrition and Dietary Supplements, 5, 27-35.

Ornish, D., Brown, S. E., Billings, J. H., Scherwitz, L. W., Armstrong, W. T., Ports, T. A., ... & Brand, R. J. (1990). Can lifestyle changes reverse coronary heart disease?: The Lifestyle Heart Trial. The Lancet, 336(8708), 129-133.

Ornish, D. & Ornish, A. (2019) 'Undo It!: How Simple Lifestyle Changes Can Reverse Most Chronic Diseases.' Ballantine Books, New York.

Ornish, D., Scherwitz, L. W., Billings, J. H., Gould, K. L., Merritt, T. A., Sparler, S., ... & Brand, R. J. (1998). Intensive lifestyle changes for reversal of coronary heart disease. Jama, 280(23), 2001-2007.

Orrego, R., Leiva, E., & Cheel, J. (2009). Inhibitory effect of three C-glycosylflavonoids from Cymbopogon citratus (Lemongrass) on human low density lipoprotein oxidation. Molecules, 14(10), 3906-3913.

Osakabe, N., Takano, H., Sanbongi, C., Yasuda, A., Yanagisawa, R., Inoue, K. I., & Yoshikawa, T. (2004). Anti-inflammatory and anti-allergic effect of rosmarinic acid (RA); inhibition of seasonal allergic rhinoconjunctivitis (SAR) and its mechanism. Biofactors, 21(1-4), 127-131.

Ostlund Jr, R. E. (2002). Phytosterols in human nutrition. Annual review of nutrition, 22(1), 533-549.

Ozgoli, G., Goli, M., & Moattar, F. (2009). Comparison of effects of ginger, mefenamic acid, and ibuprofen on pain in women with primary dysmenorrhea. The Journal of alternative and complementary medicine, 15(2), 129-132.

Pallauf, K., Giller, K., Huebbe, P., & Rimbach, G. (2013). Nutrition and healthy ageing: calorie restriction or polyphenol-rich 'MediterrAsian' diet?. Oxidative medicine and cellular longevity, 2013.

Palu, A. K., Kim, A. H., West, B. J., Deng, S., Jensen, J., & White, L. (2008). The effects of Morinda citrifolia L.(noni) on the immune system: its molecular mechanisms of action. Journal of Ethnopharmacology, 115(3), 502-506.

Panahi, Y., Khalili, N., Sahebi, E., Namazi, S., Karimian, M. S., Majeed, M., & Sahebkar, A. (2017). Antioxidant effects of curcuminoids in patients with type 2 diabetes mellitus: a randomized controlled trial. Inflammopharmacology, 25(1), 25-31.

Panahi, Y., Kianpour, P., Mohtashami, R., Jafari, R., Simental-Mendía, L. E., & Sahebkar, A. (2016). Curcumin lowers serum lipids and uric acid in subjects with nonalcoholic fatty liver disease: a randomized controlled trial. Journal of cardiovascular pharmacology, 68(3), 223-229.

Pandey, Y., Bhatt, S. S., & Debbarma, N. (2018). Watercress (Nasturtium officinale): A Potential Source of Nutraceuticals. Int. J. Curr. Microbiol. App. Sci, 7(2), 2685-2691.

Panno, M. L., Giordano, F., Rizza, P., Pellegrino, M., Zito, D., Giordano, C., ... & De Amicis, F. (2012). Bergapten induces ER depletion in breast cancer cells through SMAD4-mediated ubiquitination. Breast cancer research and treatment, 136(2), 443-455.

Paocharoen, V. (2010). The efficacy and side effects of oral Centella asiatica extract for wound healing promotion in diabetic wound patients. J Med Assoc Thai, 93(Suppl 7), S166-S170.

Park, S. Y., Kim, Y. H., Kim, Y., & Lee, S. J. (2012). Aromatic-turmerone attenuates invasion and expression of MMP-9 and COX-2 through inhibition of NF-κB activation in TPA-induced breast cancer cells. Journal of cellular biochemistry, 113(12), 3653-3662.

Pascoe, B. (2014). Dark Emu Black Seeds: Agriculture Or Accident?. Magabala Books.

Pastor, R. F., Gonzalez, E., Cassini, M. S., Pastor, I., Sauré, M., Saavedra, E., ... & Iermoli, R. H. (2016). Blueberry Extract Reduces Oxidative Stress in Patients with Metabolic Syndrome. Journal of Life Sciences, 10, 145-152.

Patel, A. V., Rojas-Vera, J., & Dacke, C. G. (2004). Therapeutic constituents and actions of Rubus species. Current medicinal chemistry, 11(11), 1501-1512.

Patterson, E., Wall, R., Fitzgerald, G. F., Ross, R. P., & Stanton, C. (2012). Health implications of high dietary omega-6 polyunsaturated fatty acids. Journal of nutrition and metabolism, 2012.

Pearson, D. A., Paglieroni, T. G., Rein, D., Wun, T., Schramm, D. D., Wang, J. F., ... & Keen, C. L. (2002). The effects of flavanol-rich cocoa and aspirin on ex vivo platelet function. Thrombosis research, 106(4), 191-197.

Pedret, A., Valls, R. M., Fernández-Castillejo, S., Catalán, Ú., Romeu, M., Giralt, M., ... & Espinel, A. (2012). Polyphenol-rich foods exhibit DNA antioxidative properties and protect the glutathione system in healthy subjects. Molecular nutrition & food research, 56(7), 1025-1033.

Pék, Z., Daood, H., Nagyné, M. G., Berki, M., Tóthné, M. M., Neményi, A., & Helyes, L. (2012). Yield and phytochemical compounds of broccoli as affected by temperature, irrigation, and foliar sulfur supplementation. HortScience, 47(11), 1646-1652.

Peou, S., Milliard-Hasting, B., & Shah, S. A. (2016). Impact of avocado-enriched diets on plasma lipoproteins: A meta-analysis. Journal of clinical lipidology, 10(1), 161-171.

Percival, S. S., Vanden Heuvel, J. P., Nieves, C. J., Montero, C., Migliaccio, A. J., & Meadors, J. (2012). Bioavailability of herbs and spices in humans as determined by ex vivo inflammatory suppression and DNA strand breaks. Journal of the American College of Nutrition, 31(4), 288-294.

Pereira, C., Li, D., & Sinclair, A. J. (2001). The alpha-linolenic acid content of green vegetables commonly available in Australia. International journal for vitamin and nutrition research, 71(4), 223-228.

Peterson, J. M., Wang, D. J., Shettigar, V., Roof, S. R., Canan, B. D., Bakkar, N., ... & Londhe, P. (2018). NF-κB inhibition rescues cardiac function by remodeling calcium genes in a Duchenne muscular dystrophy model. Nature communications, 9(1), 3431.

Phillips, K. M., Ruggio, D. M., & Ashraf-Khorassani, M. (2005). Phytosterol composition of nuts and seeds commonly consumed in the United States. Journal of agricultural and food chemistry, 53(24), 9436-9445.

PhytoHub (2017). http://phytohub.eu

Ponzo, V., Goitre, I., Fadda, M., Gambino, R., De Francesco, A., Soldati, L., ... & Bo, S. (2015). Dietary flavonoid intake and cardiovascular risk: a population-based cohort study. Journal of translational medicine, 13(1), 218.

Pawlowska, A. M., Oleszek, W., & Braca, A. (2008). Quali-quantitative analyses of flavonoids of Morus nigra L. and Morus alba L.(Moraceae) fruits. Journal of agricultural and food chemistry, 56(9), 3377-3380.

Pietrzkowski, Z., Nemzer, B., Spórna, A., Stalica, P., Tresher, W., Keller, R., ... & Wybraniec, S. (2010). Influence of betalain-rich extract on reduction of discomfort associated with osteoarthritis. New Med, 1, 12-17.

Poiroux-Gonord, F., Bidel, L. P., Fanciullino, A. L., Gautier, H., Lauri-Lopez, F., & Urban, L. (2010). Health benefits of vitamins and secondary metabolites of fruits and vegetables and prospects to increase their concentrations by agronomic approaches. Journal of Agricultural and Food Chemistry, 58(23), 12065-12082.

Pollan, M. (2008). 'In Defence of Food. An eater's manifesto.' Penguin Books.

Potter, G. A., & Burke, M. D. (2006). Salvestrols-natural products with tumour selective activity. Journal of Orthomolecular Medicine, 21(1), 34-36.

Prasad, K. N. (2015). Treat Concussion, TBI, and PTSD with Vitamins and Antioxidants. Simon and Schuster.

Prasad, S., Tyagi, A. K., Siddik, Z. H., & Aggarwal, B. B. (2017). Curcumin-Free Turmeric Exhibits Activity against Human HCT-116 Colon Tumor Xenograft: Comparison with Curcumin and Whole Turmeric. Frontiers in pharmacology, 8.

Premkumar, L. S. (2014). Transient receptor potential channels as targets for phytochemicals. ACS chemical neuroscience, 5(11), 1117-1130.

Price, J. R., Lamberton, J. A., & Culvenor, C. C. J. (1993). The Australian Phytochemical Survey: historical aspects of the CSIRO search for new drugs in Australian plants. Historical records of Australian science, 9(4), 335-356.

Procházková, D., Boušová, I., & Wilhelmová, N. (2011). Antioxidant and prooxidant properties of flavonoids. Fitoterapia, 82(4), 513-523.

Provenza, F. D., Meuret, M., & Gregorini, P. (2015). Our landscapes, our livestock, ourselves: Restoring broken linkages among plants, herbivores, and humans with diets that nourish and satiate. Appetite, 95, 500-519.

Prucksunand, C., Indrasukhsri, B., Leethochawalit, M., & Hungspreugs, K. (2001). Phase II clinical trial on effect of the long turmeric (Curcuma longa Linn) on healing of peptic ulcer. The Southeast Asian journal of tropical medicine and public health, 32(1), 208-215.

Puangsombat, K., Jirapakkul, W., & Smith, J. S. (2011). Inhibitory activity of Asian spices on heterocyclic amines formation in cooked beef patties. Journal of food science, 76(8), T174-T180.

Punyasiri, P. A. N., Abeysinghe, I. S. B., Kumar, V., Treutter, D., Duy, D., Gosch, C., ... & Fischer, T. C. (2004). Flavonoid biosynthesis in the tea plant Camellia sinensis: properties of enzymes of the prominent epicatechin and catechin pathways. Archives of Biochemistry and Biophysics, 431(1), 22-30.

Rabinkov, A., Miron, T., Mirelman, D., Wilchek, M., Glozman, S., Yavin, E., & Weiner, L. (2000). S-Allylmercaptoglutathione: the reaction product of allicin with glutathione possesses SH-modifying and antioxidant properties. Biochimica et Biophysica Acta (BBA)-Molecular Cell Research, 1499(1), 144-153.

Rafiq, S., Kaul, R., Sofi, S. A., Bashir, N., Nazir, F., & Nayik, G. A. (2016). Citrus peel as a source of functional ingredient: a review. Journal of the Saudi Society of Agricultural Sciences.

Rahal, A., Kumar, A., Singh, V., Yadav, B., Tiwari, R., Chakraborty, S., & Dhama, K. (2014). Oxidative stress, prooxidants, and antioxidants: the interplay. BioMed research international, 2014.

Rahman, K., Lowe, G. M., & Smith, S. (2016). Aged garlic extract inhibits human platelet aggregation by altering intracellular signaling and platelet shape change. The Journal of nutrition, 146(2), 410S-415S.

Rains, T. M., Agarwal, S., & Maki, K. C. (2011). Antiobesity effects of green tea catechins: a mechanistic review. The Journal of nutritional biochemistry, 22(1), 1-7.

Ramdhan, B., Chikmawati, T., & Waluyo, E. B. (2015). Ethnomedical herb from Cikondang indigenous village, district Bandung West Java Indonesia. Journal of Biodiversity and Environmental Sciences (JBES), 277-288.

Ramsden, C. E., Hibbeln, J. R., Majchrzak, S. F., & Davis, J. M. (2010). n-6 fatty acid-specific and mixed polyunsaturate dietary interventions have different effects on CHD risk: a meta-analysis of randomised controlled trials. British Journal of Nutrition, 104 (11), 1586-1600.

Read, C., & Menary, R. (2000). Analysis of the contents of oil cells in Tasmannia lanceolata (Poir.) AC Smith (Winteraceae). Annals of Botany, 86(6), 1193-1197.

Read, J., Gras, E., Sanson, G. D., Clissold, F., & Brunt, C. (2003). Does chemical defence decline more in developing leaves that become strong and tough at maturity? Australian Journal of Botany, 51(5), 489-496.

Ren, F., Reilly, K., Kerry, J. P., Gaffney, M., Hossain, M., & Rai, D. K. (2017). Higher antioxidant activity, total flavonols, and specific quercetin glucosides in two different onion (Allium cepa L.) varieties grown under organic production: results from a 6-year field study. Journal of agricultural and food chemistry, 65(25), 5122-5132.

Rendeiro, C., Rhodes, J. S., & Spencer, J. P. (2015). The mechanisms of action of flavonoids in the brain: direct versus indirect effects. Neurochemistry international, 89, 126-139.

Rensing, K. L., Reuwer, A. Q., Arsenault, B. J., von der Thüsen, J. H., Hoekstra, J. B. L., Kastelein, J. J. P., & Twickler, T. B. (2011). Reducing cardiovascular disease risk in patients with type 2 diabetes and concomitant macrovascular disease: can insulin be too much of a good thing?. Diabetes, Obesity and Metabolism, 13(12), 1073-1087.

Renzi-Hammond, L. M., Bovier, E. R., Fletcher, L. M., Miller, L. S., Mewborn, C. M., Lindbergh, C. A., ... & Hammond, B. R. (2017). Effects of a Lutein and Zeaxanthin Intervention on Cognitive Function: A Randomized, Double-Masked, Placebo-Controlled Trial of Younger Healthy Adults. Nutrients, 9(11), 1246.

Riaz, M., Ashfaq, U. A., Qasim, M., Yasmeen, E., Qamar, M. T. U., & Anwar, F. (2017). Screening of medicinal plant phytochemicals as natural antagonists of p53–MDM2 interaction to reactivate p53 functioning. Anti-Cancer Drugs, 28(9), 1032-1038.

Ribaya-Mercado, J. D., & Blumberg, J. B. (2004). Lutein and zeaxanthin and their potential roles in disease prevention. Journal of the American College of Nutrition, 23(sup6), 567S-587S.

Ried, K. (2016). Garlic Lowers Blood Pressure in Hypertensive Individuals, Regulates Serum Cholesterol, and Stimulates Immunity: An Updated Meta-analysis and Review, 2. The Journal of nutrition, 146(2), 389S-396S.

RIRDC (2014a). Focus on Anise myrtle, Syzygium anisatum. Rural Industries Research and Development Corporation, Publication 14/110.

RIRDC (2014b). Focus on Kakadu plum, Terminalia ferdinandiana. Rural Industries Research and Development Corporation, Publication 14/115.

Riso, P., Klimis-Zacas, D., Del Bo, C., Martini, D., Campolo, J., Vendrame, S., ... &

Porrini, M. (2013). Effect of a wild blueberry (Vaccinium angustifolium) drink intervention on markers of oxidative stress, inflammation and endothelial function in humans with cardiovascular risk factors. European journal of nutrition, 52(3), 949-961.

Rivlin, R. S. (2001). Historical perspective on the use of garlic. The Journal of nutrition, 131(3), 951S-954S.

Rock, K. L., & Kono, H. (2008). The inflammatory response to cell death. Annu. Rev. pathmechdis. Mech. Dis., 3, 99-126.

Rodríguez-Morató, J., Xicota, L., Fito, M., Farre, M., Dierssen, M., & de la Torre, R. (2015). Potential role of olive oil phenolic compounds in the prevention of neurodegenerative diseases. Molecules, 20(3), 4655-4680.

Roqaiya, M., Begum, W., Majeedi, S. F., & Saiyed, A. (2015). A review on traditional uses and phytochemical properties of Mimusops elengi Linn. International Journal of Herbal Medicine, 2(6), 20-23.

Rose, S. (2010). For all the tea in China. Espionage, empire and the secret formula for the world's favourite drink. Arrow Books.

Roshdy, E., Rajaratnam, V., Maitra, S., Sabry, M., Allah, A. S. A., & Al-Hendy, A. (2013). Treatment of symptomatic uterine fibroids with green tea extract: a pilot randomized controlled clinical study. International journal of women's health, 5, 477.

Rothwell JA, Pérez-Jiménez J, Neveu V, Medina-Ramon A, M'Hiri N, Garcia Lobato P, Manach C, Knox K, Eisner R, Wishart D, Scalbert A. (2013) Phenol-Explorer 3.0: a major update of the Phenol-Explorer database to incorporate data on the effects of food processing on polyphenol content. Database, 10.1093/database/bat070.

Rupp, R. (2011). 'How Carrots Won the Trojan war. Curious (but true) stories of common vegetables.' Storey Publishing, MASS USA.

Rusznyak, S. T., & Szent-Györgyi, A. (1936). Vitamin P: flavonols as vitamins. Nature, 138 (3479): 27.

Sacks, F. M., & Campos, H. (2010). Dietary therapy in hypertension. New England journal of medicine, 362(22), 2102-2112.

Sacks, F. M., Obarzanek, E., Windhauser, M. M., Svetkey, L. P., Vollmer, W. M., McCullough, M., ... & Evans, M. A. (1995). Rationale and design of the Dietary Approaches to Stop Hypertension trial (DASH): a multicenter controlled-feeding study of dietary patterns to lower blood pressure. Annals of epidemiology, 5(2), 108-118.

Sacks, F. M., Svetkey, L. P., Vollmer, W. M., Appel, L. J., Bray, G. A., Harsha, D., ... & Karanja, N. (2001). Effects on blood pressure of reduced dietary sodium and the Dietary Approaches to Stop Hypertension (DASH) diet. New England journal of medicine, 344(1), 3-10.

Sakulnarmrat, K. (2012). Potential health properties of selected commercially grown native Australian herbs and fruits. PhD Thesis, University of New South Wales.

Sakulnarmrat, K., Fenech, M., Thomas, P., & Konczak, I. (2013). Cytoprotective and pro-apoptotic activities of native Australian herbs polyphenolic-rich extracts. Food chemistry, 136(1), 9-17.

Sakulnarmrat, K., Srzednicki, G., & Konczak, I. (2015). Bioprospecting Davidson's plum and quandong: Cytoprotective and proapoptotic activities. LWT-Food

Science and Technology, 61(2), 622-629.

Salas-Salvadó, J., Bulló, M., Babio, N., Martínez-González, M. Á., Ibarrola-Jurado, N., Basora, J., ... & Ruiz-Gutiérrez, V. (2010). Reduction in the incidence of type 2-diabetes with the Mediterranean diet: results of the PREDIMED-Reus nutrition intervention randomized trial. Diabetes care.

Salazar, R., Arámbula-Villa, G., Hidalgo, F. J., & Zamora, R. (2014). Structural characteristics that determine the inhibitory role of phenolic compounds on 2-amino-1-methyl-6-phenylimidazo [4, 5-b] pyridine (PhIP) formation. Food chemistry, 151, 480-486.

Saldanha, S. N., Kala, R., & Tollefsbol, T. O. (2014). Molecular mechanisms for inhibition of colon cancer cells by combined epigenetic-modulating epigallocatechin gallate and sodium butyrate. Experimental cell research, 324(1), 40-53.

Salvamani, S., Gunasekaran, B., Shaharuddin, N. A., Ahmad, S. A., & Shukor, M. Y. (2014). Antiartherosclerotic effects of plant flavonoids. BioMed Research International, 2014.

Sambhav, J., Rohit, R., Ankit Raj, U., & Garima, M. (2014). Curcuma longa in the management of inflammatory diseases—A review. Int Ayur Med J, 2(1), 34-40.

Sandur, S. K., Pandey, M. K., Sung, B., Ahn, K. S., Murakami, A., Sethi, G., ... & Aggarwal, B. B. (2007). Curcumin, demethoxycurcumin, bisdemethoxycurcumin, tetrahydrocurcumin and turmerones differentially regulate anti-inflammatory and anti-proliferative responses through a ROS-independent mechanism. Carcinogenesis, 28(8), 1765-1773.

Saud, S. M., Li, W., Gray, Z., Matter, M. S., Colburn, N. H., Young, M. R., & Kim, Y. S. (2016). Diallyl disulfide (DADS), a constituent of garlic, inactivates NF-κB and prevents colitis-induced colorectal cancer by inhibiting GSK-3β. Cancer Prevention Research, 9(7), 607-615.

Sayeed, M. A., Bracci, M., Lucarini, G., Lazzarini, R., Di Primio, R., & Santarelli, L. (2017). Regulation of microRNA using promising dietary phytochemicals: Possible preventive and treatment option of malignant mesothelioma. Biomedicine & Pharmacotherapy, 94, 1197-1224.

Sayem, A. S. M., Arya, A., Karimian, H., Krishnasamy, N., Ashok Hasamnis, A., & Hossain, C. F. (2018). Action of Phytochemicals on Insulin Signaling Pathways Accelerating Glucose Transporter (GLUT4) Protein Translocation. Molecules, 23(2), 258.

Schaefer, B. A. (2012). Salvestrols: Nature's Defence Against Cancer: Linking Diet and Cancer. Clinical Intelligence Corporation.

Schaefer, B. A., Dooner, C., Danny Burke, M., & Potter, G. A. (2010). Nutrition and cancer: further case studies involving Salvestrol. Journal of Orthomolecular Medicine, 25(1), 17.

Schlemmer, U., Frølich, W., Prieto, R. M., & Grases, F. (2009). Phytate in foods and significance for humans: food sources, intake, processing, bioavailability, protective role and analysis. Molecular nutrition & food research, 53(S2).

Scholey, A. B., Tildesley, N. T., Ballard, C. G., Wesnes, K. A., Tasker, A., Perry, E. K., & Kennedy, D. O. (2008). An extract of Salvia (sage) with anticholinesterase properties improves memory and attention in healthy older volunteers. Psychopharmacology, 198(1), 127-139.

Schonhof, I., Blankenburg, D., Müller, S., & Krumbein, A. (2007). Sulfur and nitrogen supply influence growth, product appearance, and glucosinolate concentration of broccoli. Journal of Plant Nutrition and Soil Science, 170(1), 65-72.

Schulick, P. (2012). 'Ginger: common spice & wonder drug'. Kalindi Press, Chino Valley Arizona pp 140.

Scoditti, E., Calabriso, N., Massaro, M., Pellegrino, M., Storelli, C., Martines, G., ... & Carluccio, M. A. (2012). Mediterranean diet polyphenols reduce inflammatory angiogenesis through MMP-9 and COX-2 inhibition in human vascular endo-thelial cells: a potentially protective mechanism in atherosclerotic vascular disease and cancer. Archives of biochemistry and biophysics, 527(2), 81-89.

Semple, S. J., Reynolds, G. D., O'leary, M. C., & Flower, R. L. P. (1998). Screening of Australian medicinal plants for antiviral activity. Journal of Ethnopharmacology, 60(2), 163-172.

Seyfried, T. N. (2015). Cancer as a mitochondrial metabolic disease. Frontiers in cell and developmental biology, 3.

Serafini, M., Ghiselli, A., & Ferro-Luzzi, A. (1996). In vivo antioxidant effect of green and black tea in man. European journal of clinical nutrition, 50(1), 28-32.

Shahzad, N., Khan, W., Shadab, M. D., Ali, A., Saluja, S. S., Sharma, S., ... & Afify, M. A. (2017). Phytosterols as a natural anticancer agent: Current status and future perspective. Biomedicine & Pharmacotherapy, 88, 786-794.

Sharangi, A. B. (2009). Medicinal and therapeutic potentialities of tea (Camellia sinensis L.)–A review. Food Research International, 42(5-6), 529-535.

Sharma, R. A., Euden, S. A., Platton, S. L., Cooke, D. N., Shafayat, A., Hewitt, H. R., ... & Pirmohamed, M. (2004). Phase I clinical trial of oral curcumin: biomark-ers of systemic activity and compliance. Clinical Cancer Research, 10(20), 6847-6854.

Shatzker M. (2015) *The Dorito Effect. The surprising new truth about food and flavour*. Simon and Schuster, New York.

Shipard I. (2003). 'How can I use herbs in my daily life? Over 500 herbs, spices and edible plants: An Australian practical guide to growing culinary and medicinal herbs'. Publihsed by David Stewart. Printed by Queensland Complete Printing Services, Nambour Queensland.

Shishodia, S., Amin, H. M., Lai, R., & Aggarwal, B. B. (2005). Curcumin (diferuloylmeth-ane) inhibits constitutive NF-κB activation, induces G1/S arrest, suppresses proliferation, and induces apoptosis in mantle cell lymphoma. Biochemical pharmacology, 70(5), 700-713.

Shoba, G., Joy, D., Joseph, T., Majeed, M., Rajendran, R., & Srinivas, P. S. S. R. (1998). Influence of piperine on the pharmacokinetics of curcumin in animals and human volunteers. Planta medica, 64(04), 353-356.

Silva, S., Bronze, M. R., Figueira, M. E., Siwy, J., Mischak, H., Combet, E., & Mullen, W. (2015). Impact of a 6-wk olive oil supplementation in healthy adults on urinary proteomic biomarkers of coronary artery disease, chronic kidney disease, and diabetes (types 1 and 2): a randomized, parallel, controlled, double-blind study. The American journal of clinical nutrition, 101(1), 44-54.

Singh, B., Singh, J. P., Kaur, A., & Singh, N. (2016). Bioactive compounds in banana and their associated health benefits–A review. Food Chemistry, 206, 1-11.

Singh, K., Connors, S. L., Macklin, E. A., Smith, K. D., Fahey, J. W., Talalay, P., & Zimmerman, A. W. (2014). Sulforaphane treatment of autism spectrum disorder (ASD). Proceedings of the National Academy of Sciences, 111(43),

15550-15555.

Sinha, R., Anderson, D. E., McDonald, S. S., & Greenwald, P. (2003). Cancer risk and diet in India. Journal of postgraduate medicine, 49(3), 222.

Sinkovic, A., Suran, D., Lokar, L., Fliser, E., Skerget, M., Novak, Z., & Knez, Z. (2011). Rosemary extracts improve flow-mediated dilatation of the brachial artery and plasma PAI-1 activity in healthy young volunteers. Phytotherapy research, 25(3), 402-407.

Slimestad, R., & Verheul, M. (2009). Review of flavonoids and other phenolics from fruits of different tomato (Lycopersicon esculentum Mill.) cultivars. Journal of the Science of Food and Agriculture, 89(8), 1255-1270.

Somerset, S. M., & Johannot, L. (2008). Dietary flavonoid sources in Australian adults. Nutrition and cancer, 60(4), 442-449.

Song, Y., Manson, J. E., Buring, J. E., Sesso, H. D., & Liu, S. (2005). Associations of dietary flavonoids with risk of type 2 diabetes, and markers of insulin resistance and systemic inflammation in women: a prospective study and cross-sectional analysis. Journal of the American College of Nutrition, 24(5), 376-384.

Speciale, G., Jin, Y., Davies, G. J., Williams, S. J., & Goddard-Borger, E. D. (2016). YihQ is a sulfoquinovosidase that cleaves sulfoquinovosyl diacylglyceride sulfolipids. Nature chemical biology, 12(4), 215.

Spiller, G. A., Jenkins, D. A., Bosello, O., Gates, J. E., Cragen, L. N., & Bruce, B. (1998). Nuts and plasma lipids: an almond-based diet lowers LDL-C while preserving HDL-C. Journal of the American College of Nutrition, 17(3), 285-290.

Stuart J. M. and Hardman W. (1865). 'The Journals of John McDouall Stuart during the years 1858, 1859, 1860, 1861, & 1862, when he fixed the centre of the continent and successfully crossed it from sea to sea. Edited from Mr. Stuart's Manuscript.' Second Edition. Saunders, Otley and Co, London.

Sugimura, T., M. Nagao, T. Kawachi, M. Honda, T. Yahagi, Y. Seino, S. Stao, N. Matsukura, T. Matsushima, A. Shirai, M. Sawamura and H. Matsumoto (1977). Mutagen-carcinogens in food, with special reference to highly mutagenic pyrolytic products in broiled foods, in: H.H. Hiatt, J.D. Watson and J.A. Winstein _Eds., Origins of Human Cancer, Book C, Cold Spring Harbor Laboratory, Cold Spring Harbor, NY, pp. 1561–1577.

Sugimura, T. (1997). Overview of carcinogenic heterocyclic amines. Mutation Research. Fundamental and Molecular Mechanisms of Mutagenesis, 376(1), 211-219.

Sultana, B., & Anwar, F. (2008). Flavonols (kaempeferol, quercetin, myricetin) contents of selected fruits, vegetables and medicinal plants. Food Chemistry, 108(3), 879-884.

Sumner, M. D., Elliott-Eller, M., Weidner, G., Daubenmier, J. J., Chew, M. H., Marlin, R., ... & Ornish, D. (2005). Effects of pomegranate juice consumption on myocardial perfusion in patients with coronary heart disease. The American journal of cardiology, 96(6), 810-814.

Sun, W., Frost, B., & Liu, J. (2017). Oleuropein, unexpected benefits! Oncotarget, 8 (11), 17409.

Sun Y., Liu B., Snetselaar L. G, Robinson J. G, Wallace R. B, Peterson L. L et al. Association of fried food consumption with all cause, cardiovascular, and cancer mortality: prospective cohort study BMJ 2019; 364 :k5420

Surh, Y. J. (2011). Xenohormesis mechanisms underlying chemopreventive effects of some dietary phytochemicals. Annals of the New York Academy of Sciences, 1229(1), 1-6.

Surh, Y. J. (2011). Xenohormesis mechanisms underlying chemopreventive effects of some dietary phytochemicals. Annals of the New York Academy of Sciences, 1229(1), 1-6.

Symonds, E. L., Konczak, I., & Fenech, M. (2013). The Australian fruit Illawarra plum (Podocarpus elatus Endl., Podocarpaceae) inhibits telomerase, increases histone deacetylase activity and decreases proliferation of colon cancer cells. British Journal of Nutrition, 109(12), 2117-2125.

Szent-Gyorgyi A. (1937) Oxidation, energy transfer, and vitamins. 1937 Nobel Prize for Medicine acceptance Lecture.

Takahama, U., & Hirota, S. (2018). Interactions of flavonoids with α-amylase and starch slowing down its digestion. Food & function, 9, 677-687.

Tan, A. C., Konczak, I., Ramzan, I., & Sze, D. M. Y. (2011a). Antioxidant and cyto-protective activities of native Australian fruit polyphenols. Food research international, 44(7), 2034-2040.

Tan, A. C., Konczak, I., Ramzan, I., Zabaras, D., & Sze, D. M. Y. (2011b). Potential antioxidant, antiinflammatory, and proapoptotic anticancer activities of Kakadu plum and Illawarra plum polyphenolic fractions. Nutrition and cancer, 63(7), 1074-1084.

Tanaka, S., Haruma, K., Yoshihara, M., Kajiyama, G., Kira, K., Amagase, H., & Chayama, K. (2006). Aged garlic extract has potential suppressive effect on colorectal adenomas in humans. The Journal of nutrition, 136(3), 821S-826S.

Tang, K. S., Konczak, I., & Zhao, J. (2016). Identification and quantification of phenolics in Australian native mint (Mentha australis R. Br.). Food chemistry, 192, 698-705.

Tang, M., & Taghibiglou, C. (2017). The Mechanisms of Action of Curcumin in Alzheimer's Disease. Journal of Alzheimer's Disease, (Preprint), 1-14.

Tang, L., Zirpoli, G. R., Guru, K., Moysich, K. B., Zhang, Y., Ambrosone, C. B., & McCann, S. E. (2010). Intake of cruciferous vegetables modifies bladder cancer survival. Cancer Epidemiology and Prevention Biomarkers, 19(7), 1806-1811.

Tang, Y., & Tsao, R. (2017). Phytochemicals in quinoa and amaranth grains and their antioxidant, anti-inflammatory, and potential health beneficial effects: a review. Molecular nutrition & food research, 61(7), 1600767.

Taqvi, S. I. H., Shah, A. J., & Gilani, A. H. (2008). Blood pressure lowering and vaso-modulator effects of piperine. Journal of cardiovascular pharmacology, 52(5), 452-458.

Tarazona-Díaz, M. P., Alacid, F., Carrasco, M., Martínez, I., & Aguayo, E. (2013). Watermelon juice: potential functional drink for sore muscle relief in athletes. Journal of agricultural and food chemistry, 61(31), 7522-7528.

Tardío, J., Pardo-de-Santayana, M., & Morales, R. (2006). Ethnobotanical review of wild edible plants in Spain. Botanical Journal of the Linnean Society, 152(1), 27-71.

Telfer, A. (2002). What is β−carotene doing in the photosystem II reaction centre?. Philosophical Transactions of the Royal Society of London B: Biological Sciences, 357(1426), 1431-1440.

Terés, S., Barceló-Coblijn, G., Benet, M., Alvarez, R., Bressani, R., Halver, J. E., & Escriba, P. V. (2008). Oleic acid content is responsible for the reduction in blood pressure induced by olive oil. Proceedings of the National Academy of Sciences.

Teruya, T., Chaleckis, R., Takada, J., Yanagida, M., & Kondoh, H. (2019). Diverse Metabolic Reactions Activated During 58-hr Fasting are Revealed by Non-Targeted Metabolomic Analysis of Human Blood. Scientific Reports 9: 854.

Tewksbury, J. J., Reagan, K. M., Machnicki, N. J., Carlo, T. A., Haak, D. C., Peñaloza, A. L. C., & Levey, D. J. (2008). Evolutionary ecology of pungency in wild chilies. Proceedings of the National Academy of Sciences, 105(33), 11808-11811.

Theunissen, S., Balestra, C., Boutros, A., De Bels, D., Guerrero, F., & Germonpré, P. (2015). The effect of pre-dive ingestion of dark chocolate on endothelial function after a scuba dive. Diving Hyperb Med, 45(1), 4-9.

Thomson, M., Corbin, R., & Leung, L. (2014). Effects of ginger for nausea and vomiting in early pregnancy: a meta-analysis. The Journal of the American Board of Family Medicine, 27(1), 115-122.

Tieman, D., Zhu, G., Resende, M. F., Lin, T., Nguyen, C., Bies, D., ... & Ikeda, H. (2017). A chemical genetic roadmap to improved tomato flavor. Science, 355(6323), 391-394.

Tildesley, N. T. J., Kennedy, D. O., Perry, E. K., Ballard, C. G., Wesnes, K. A., & Scholey, A. B. (2005). Positive modulation of mood and cognitive performance following administration of acute doses of Salvia lavandulaefolia essential oil to healthy young volunteers. Physiology & behavior, 83(5), 699-709.

Tili, E., & Michaille, J. J. (2016). Promiscuous Effects of Some Phenolic Natural Products on Inflammation at Least in Part Arise from Their Ability to Modulate the Expression of Global Regulators, Namely microRNAs. Molecules, 21(9), 1263.

Tiwari, S., Singh, S., Patwardhan, K., Gehlot, S., & Gambhir, I. S. (2008). Effect of Centella asiatica on mild cognitive impairment (MCI) and other common age-related clinical problems. Digest Journal of Nanomaterials and Biostructures, 3(4), 215-220.

Tolhurst, P., Lindberg, R., Calder, R., & de Courten, M. (2016). 'Australia's health tracker 2016: A report card on preventable chronic diseases, conditions and their risk factors: Tracking progress for a healthier Australia by 2025.' Melbourne: The Australian Health Policy Collaboration.

Toden, S., & Goel, A. (2017). The Holy Grail of Curcumin and its Efficacy in Various Diseases: Is Bioavailability Truly a Big Concern?. Journal of Restorative Medicine, 6(1), 27-36.

Tomás-Barberán, F. A., González-Sarrías, A., García-Villalba, R., Núñez-Sánchez, M. A., Selma, M. V., García-Conesa, M. T., & Espín, J. C. (2017). Urolithins, the rescue of 'old' metabolites to understand a 'new' concept: Metabotypes as a nexus among phenolic metabolism, microbiota dysbiosis, and host health status. Molecular nutrition & food research, 61(1).

Törrönen, R., Sarkkinen, E., Niskanen, T., Tapola, N., Kilpi, K., & Niskanen, L. (2012). Postprandial glucose, insulin and glucagon-like peptide 1 responses to sucrose ingested with berries in healthy subjects. British journal of nutrition, 107(10), 1445-1451.

Toussaint, J. P., Smith, F. A., & Smith, S. E. (2007). Arbuscular mycorrhizal fungi can induce the production of phytochemicals in sweet basil irrespective of phosphorus nutrition. Mycorrhiza, 17(4), 291-297.

Toussirot, É., & Wendling, D. (2007). The use of TNF-α blocking agents in rheumatoid arthritis: an update. Expert opinion on pharmacotherapy, 8(13), 2089-2107.

Traynor S. and Breen R. (2010). John McDouall Stuart's 1860 Expedition a 'Natural' History. *Alice Springs Field Naturalist Club Newsletter* April 2010, pages 3 - 4.

Tsujiyama, I., Mubassara, S., Aoshima, H., & Hossain, S. J. (2013). Anti-histamine release and anti-inflammatory activities of aqueous extracts of citrus fruits peels. Oriental Pharmacy and Experimental Medicine, 13(3), 175-180.

Tzounis, X., Rodriguez-Mateos, A., Vulevic, J., Gibson, G. R., Kwik-Uribe, C., & Spencer, J. P. (2011). Prebiotic evaluation of cocoa-derived flavanols in healthy humans by using a randomized, controlled, double-blind, crossover intervention study. The American journal of clinical nutrition, 93(1), 62-72.

USDA (2018) U.S. Department of Agriculture, Agricultural Research Service. 2018. USDA National Nutrient Database for Standard Reference, Release . Nutrient Data Laboratory Home Page, http://www.ars.usda.gov/nutrientdata Cited 21 July 2018.

Van Cauwenberghe, C., Vandendriessche, C., Libert, C., & Vandenbroucke, R. E. (2016). Caloric restriction: beneficial effects on brain aging and Alzheimer's disease. Mammalian genome, 27(7-8), 300-319.

Treutter, D. (2006). Significance of flavonoids in plant resistance: a review. Environmental Chemistry Letters, 4(3), 147-157.

Villanueva, C., & Giulivi, C. (2010). Subcellular and cellular locations of nitric oxide synthase isoforms as determinants of health and disease. Free Radical Biology and Medicine, 49(3), 307-316.

Van De Wier, B., Koek, G. H., Bast, A., & Haenen, G. R. (2017). The potential of flavonoids in the treatment of non-alcoholic fatty liver disease. Critical reviews in food science and nutrition, 57(4), 834-855.

Van Etten, H. D., Mansfield, J. W., Bailey, J. A., & Farmer, E. E. (1994). Two Classes of Plant Antibiotics: Phytoalexins versus' Phytoanticipins'. The Plant Cell, 6(9), 1191.

Vane, J. R. (1971). Inhibition of prostaglandin synthesis as a mechanism of action for aspirin-like drugs. Nature (New Biology Archive), 231(25), 232-235.

Vane, J. R. & Botting R. M. (2003). The mechanism of action of aspirin. Thrombosis research, 110(5), 255-258.

Vauzour, D., Rodriguez-Mateos, A., Corona, G., Oruna-Concha, M. J., & Spencer, J. P. (2010). Polyphenols and human health: prevention of disease and mechanisms of action. Nutrients, 2(11), 1106-1131.

Vendrame, S., Guglielmetti, S., Riso, P., Arioli, S., Klimis-Zacas, D., & Porrini, M. (2011). Six-week consumption of a wild blueberry powder drink increases bifidobacteria in the human gut. Journal of agricultural and food chemistry, 59(24), 12815-12820.

Verma, S., & Kumar, V. (2017). Pharmacological profile of turmeric oil: A review. Lekovite sirovine, 35, 3-21.

Vennavaram, R. R. (2007). Investigation of chemical components and pharmaceutical potential of Carpobrotus species (Doctoral dissertation, University of Tasmania).

Vilela, C., Santos, S. A., Villaverde, J. J., Oliveira, L., Nunes, A., Cordeiro, N., ... &

Silvestre, A. J. (2014). Lipophilic phytochemicals from banana fruits of several Musa species. Food chemistry, 162, 247-252.

Vincent A. (2010). The Bush Tomato Handbook. Ninti One Limited 2010.

Virk-Baker, M. K., Nagy, T. R., Barnes, S., & Groopman, J. (2014). Dietary acrylamide and human cancer: a systematic review of literature. Nutrition and cancer, 66(5), 774-790.

Visioli, F., Borsani, L., & Galli, C. (2000). Diet and prevention of coronary heart disease: the potential role of phytochemicals. Cardiovascular Research, 47(3), 419-425.

Volkow, N. D., Wang, G. J., Logan, J., Alexoff, D., Fowler, J. S., Thanos, P. K., ... & Tomasi, D. (2015). Caffeine increases striatal dopamine D 2/D 3 receptor availability in the human brain. Translational psychiatry, 5(4), e549.

Vu, H. T., Robman, L., Hodge, A., McCarty, C. A., & Taylor, H. R. (2006). Lutein and zeaxanthin and the risk of cataract: the Melbourne visual impairment project. Investigative ophthalmology & visual science, 47(9), 3783-3786.

Vuong, Q. V., Hirun, S., Chuen, T. L., Goldsmith, C. D., Bowyer, M. C., Chalmers, A. C., ... & Scarlett, C. J. (2014). Physicochemical composition, antioxidant and anti-proliferative capacity of a lilly pilly (Syzygium paniculatum) extract. Journal of Herbal Medicine, 4(3), 134-140.

Wahls T. and Adamson E. (2017). 'The Wahls Protocol. How I beat progressive MS using Paleo principles and functional medicine.' Vermilion, London.

Wan, Y., Vinson, J. A., Etherton, T. D., Proch, J., Lazarus, S. A., & Kris-Etherton, P. M. (2001). Effects of cocoa powder and dark chocolate on LDL oxidative susceptibility and prostaglandin concentrations in humans. The American journal of clinical nutrition, 74(5), 596-602.

Wang, P., Aronson, W. J., Huang, M., Zhang, Y., Lee, R. P., Heber, D., & Henning, S. M. (2010). Green tea polyphenols and metabolites in prostatectomy tissue: implications for cancer prevention. Cancer Prevention Research, 3(8), 985-993.

Wang, M. Y., Lutfiyya, M. N., Weidenbacher-Hoper, V., Anderson, G., Su, C. X., & West, B. J. (2009). Antioxidant activity of noni juice in heavy smokers. Chemistry Central Journal, 3(1), 13.Wang, X., Ouyang, Y., Liu, J., Zhu, M., Zhao, G., Bao, W., & Hu, F. B. (2014). Fruit and vegetable consumption and mortality from all causes, cardiovascular disease, and cancer: systematic review and dose-response meta-analysis of prospective cohort studies. Bmj, 349, g4490.

Wangchuk, P. (2014). Phytochemical analysis, bioassays and the identification of drug lead compounds from seven Bhutanese medicinal plants.Doctor of Philosophy Thesis, School of Chemistry, University of Wollongong, New South Wales.

Watson, A. W., Haskell-Ramsay, C. F., Kennedy, D. O., Cooney, J. M., Trower, T., & Scheepens, A. (2015). Acute supplementation with blackcurrant extracts modulates cognitive functioning and inhibits monoamine oxidase-B in healthy young adults. Journal of Functional Foods, 17, 524-539.

Wattanathorn, J., Mator, L., Muchimapura, S., Tongun, T., Pasuriwong, O., Piyawatkul, N., ... & Singkhoraard, J. (2008). Positive modulation of cognition and mood in the healthy elderly volunteer following the administration of Centella asiatica. Journal of ethnopharmacology, 116(2), 325-332.

Webster, S. (2017). Grow: Full of Beans. ABC Organic Gardener, Nov/Dec 2017: 30-35.

Wedick, N. M., Pan, A., Cassidy, A., Rimm, E. B., Sampson, L., Rosner, B., ... & van

Dam, R. M. (2012). Dietary flavonoid intakes and risk of type 2 diabetes in US men and women−. The American journal of clinical nutrition, 95(4), 925-933.

Weisburger, J. H. (2002). Comments on the history and importance of aromatic and heterocyclic amines in public health. Mutation Research. Fundamental and Molecular Mechanisms of Mutagenesis, 506, 9-20.

Welch, A. A., Shakya-Shrestha, S., Lentjes, M. A., Wareham, N. J., & Khaw, K. T. (2010). Dietary intake and status of n−3 polyunsaturated fatty acids in a population of fish-eating and non-fish-eating meat-eaters, vegetarians, and vegans and the precursor-product ratio of α-linolenic acid to long-chain n−3 polyunsaturated fatty acids: results from the EPIC-Norfolk cohort−. The American journal of clinical nutrition, 92(5), 1040-1051.

Welsh, E. J., Bara, A., Barley, E., & Cates, C. J. (2010). Caffeine for asthma. The Cochrane Library.

Whyte, A. R., Schafer, G., & Williams, C. M. (2016). Cognitive effects following acute wild blueberry supplementation in 7-to 10-year-old children. European journal of nutrition, 55(6), 2151-2162.

Wien, M., Haddad, E., Oda, K., & Sabaté, J. (2013). A randomized 3x3 crossover study to evaluate the effect of Hass avocado intake on post-ingestive satiety, glucose and insulin levels, and subsequent energy intake in overweight adults. Nutrition journal, 12(1), 155.

Wigler, I., Grotto, I., Caspi, D., & Yaron, M. (2003). The effects of Zintona EC (a ginger extract) on symptomatic gonarthritis. Osteoarthritis and cartilage, 11(11), 783-789.

Wilkinson D. (2015). Can food be medicine against cancer?: a healthy handbook that combines science, medicine and not-so-common sense. Inspiring Publishers, Calwell, ACT .

Willcox, D. C., Scapagnini, G., & Willcox, B. J. (2014). Healthy aging diets other than the Mediterranean: a focus on the Okinawan diet. Mechanisms of ageing and development, 136, 148-162.

Willcox, B. J., & Willcox, D. C. (2014). Caloric Restriction, CR Mimetics, and Healthy Aging in Okinawa: Controversies and Clinical Implications. Current opinion in clinical nutrition and metabolic care, 17(1), 51.

Willcox, B. J., Willcox, C. D., & Suzuki, M. (2013). The Okinawa Way: The four-week fitness, diet and lifestyle plan to reverse the symptoms of aging. Penguin, Random House UK.

Williams, C. J. (2013). Medicinal plants in Australia Volume 4: An Antipodean Apothecary. Rosenberg Publishing.

Williamson, G., & Clifford, M. N. (2010). Colonic metabolites of berry polyphenols: the missing link to biological activity?. British Journal of Nutrition, 104(S3), S48-S66.

Wilson, L. F., Antonsson, A., Green, A. C., Jordan, S. J., Kendall, B. J., Nagle, C. M., ... & Whiteman, D. C. (2018). How many cancer cases and deaths are potentially preventable? Estimates for Australia in 2013. International journal of cancer, 142(4), 691-701.

Winters, N., & Kelley, J. H. (2017). The Metabolic Approach to Cancer: Integrating Deep Nutrition, the Ketogenic Diet, and Nontoxic Bio-Individualized Therapies. Chelsea Green Publishing.

Wium-Andersen, M. K., Ørsted, D. D., Nielsen, S. F., & Nordestgaard, B. G. (2013).

Elevated C-reactive protein levels, psychological distress, and depression in 73 131 individuals. JAMA psychiatry, 70(2), 176-184.

Wohlmuth, H., Deseo, M. A., Brushett, D. J., MacFarlane, G., Waterman, P. G., Stevenson, L. M., & Leach, D. N. (2007). Biological activity and novel cytotoxic curcuminoid from Pleuranthodium racemigerum—An Australian Zingiberaceae. Planta Medica, 73(09), P_396.

Wohlmuth, H 2008, 'Phytochemistry and pharmacology of plants from the ginger family, Zingiberaceae', PhD thesis, Southern Cross University, Lismore, NSW.

Woodward, P. (2014). Grow your own herbal remedies. Hyland House Publishing, Mebourne.

World Health Organization (2002). The world health report 2002: reducing risks, promoting healthy life. World Health Organization.

World health statistics 2017: monitoring health for the SDGs, Sustainable Development Goals. Geneva: World Health Organization; 2017. Licence: CC BY-NC-SA 3.0 IGO.

Wright, G. A., Baker, D. D., Palmer, M. J., Stabler, D., Mustard, J. A., Power, E. F., Borland A. M. and Stevenson, P. C. (2013). Caffeine in floral nectar enhances a pollinator's memory of reward. Science, 339(6124), 1202-1204.

Wu, A., Noble, E. E., Tyagi, E., Ying, Z., Zhuang, Y., & Gomez-Pinilla, F. (2015). Curcumin boosts DHA in the brain: Implications for the prevention of anxiety disorders. Biochimica et Biophysica Acta (BBA)-Molecular Basis of Disease, 1852(5), 951-961.

Wu, A., Ying, Z., & Gomez-Pinilla, F. (2004). Dietary omega-3 fatty acids normalize BDNF levels, reduce oxidative damage, and counteract learning disability after traumatic brain injury in rats. Journal of neurotrauma, 21(10), 1457-1467.

Wu, A., Ying, Z., & Gomez-Pinilla, F. (2006). Dietary curcumin counteracts the outcome of traumatic brain injury on oxidative stress, synaptic plasticity, and cognition. Experimental neurology, 197(2), 309-317.

Wu, L., Wang, Z., Zhu, J., Murad, A. L., Prokop, L. J., & Murad, M. H. (2015). Nut consumption and risk of cancer and type 2 diabetes: a systematic review and meta-analysis. Nutrition reviews, 73(7), 409-425.

Wurm, P. A. S., Campbell, L. C., Batten, G. D., & Bellairs, S. M. (2012). Australian native rice: a new sustainable wild food enterprise. Rural Industries Research and Development Corporation (RIRDC): Barton, Australia.

Xia, E., He, X., Li, H., Wu, S., Li, S. and Deng, G., Biological Activities of Polyphenols from Grapes. Chapter 5. pp 47 - 58. IN: Watson, R. R., Preedy, V. R., & Zibadi, S. (Eds.). (2013). Polyphenols in human health and disease. Academic Press.

Yadav, D., Yadav, S. K., Khar, R. K., Mujeeb, M., & Akhtar, M. (2013). Turmeric (Curcuma longa L.): A promising spice for phytochemical and pharmacological activities. International Journal of Green Pharmacy (IJGP), 7(2).

Yaffe, P. B., Power Coombs, M. R., Doucette, C. D., Walsh, M., & Hoskin, D. W. (2015). Piperine, an alkaloid from black pepper, inhibits growth of human colon cancer cells via G1 arrest and apoptosis triggered by endoplasmic reticulum stress. Molecular carcinogenesis, 54(10), 1070-1085.

Yi, L., Ma, S., & Ren, D. (2017). Phytochemistry and bioactivity of Citrus flavonoids: a focus on antioxidant, anti-inflammatory, anticancer and cardiovascular protection activities. Phytochemistry Reviews, 16(3), 479-511.

Yoon, H., & Liu, R. H. (2007). Effect of selected phytochemicals and apple extracts on NF-κB activation in human breast cancer MCF-7 cells. Journal of agricultural and food chemistry, 55(8), 3167-3173.

Yoshioka, M., St-Pierre, S., Drapeau, V., Dionne, I., Doucet, E., Suzuki, M., & Tremblay, A. (1999). Effects of red pepper on appetite and energy intake. British Journal of Nutrition, 82(2), 115-123.

Yu, E., Rimm, E., Qi, L., Rexrode, K., Albert, C. M., Sun, Q., ... & Manson, J. E. (2016). Diet, lifestyle, biomarkers, genetic factors, and risk of cardiovascular disease in the nurses' health studies. American journal of public health, 106(9), 1616-1623. Zainol, M. K., Abd-Hamid, A., Yusof, S., & Muse, R. (2003). Antioxidative activity and total phenolic compounds of leaf, root and petiole of four accessions of Centella asiatica (L.) Urban. Food Chemistry, 81(4), 575-581.

Zhan, G., Pan, L., Tu, K., & Jiao, S. (2016). Antitumor, Antioxidant, and Nitrite Scavenging Effects of Chinese Water Chestnut (Eleocharis dulcis) Peel Flavonoids. Journal of food science, 81(10).

Zhang, B., Tieman, D. M., Jiao, C., Xu, Y., Chen, K., Fe, Z., ... & Klee, H. J. (2016). Chilling-induced tomato flavor loss is associated with altered volatile synthesis and transient changes in DNA methylation. Proceedings of the National Academy of Sciences, 113(44), 12580-12585.

Zhang, F., Thakur, K., Hu, F., Zhang, J. G., & Wei, Z. J. (2017). Cross-talk between 10-gingerol and its anti-cancerous potential: a recent update. Food & Function, 8(8), 2635-2649.

Zhang, J. M., & An, J. (2007). Cytokines, inflammation and pain. International anesthesiology clinics, 45(2), 27.

Zhang, K., Han, E. S., Dellinger, T. H., Lu, J., Nam, S., Anderson, R. A., ... & Wen, W. (2017). Cinnamon extract reduces VEGF expression via suppressing HIF-1α gene expression and inhibits tumor growth in mice. Molecular carcinogenesis, 56(2), 436-446.

Zhang, Q., Liu, M., & Ruan, J. (2017). Metabolomics analysis reveals the metabolic and functional roles of flavonoids in light-sensitive tea leaves. BMC plant biology, 17(1), 64.

Zhang, W., Han, F., He, J., & Duan, C. (2008). HPLC-DAD-ESI-MS/MS Analysis and Antioxidant Activities of Nonanthocyanin Phenolics in Mulberry (Morus alba L.). Journal of food science, 73(6).

Zhong, L., Bornman, J. F., Wu, G., Hornoff, A., Dovi, K. A. P., Hayder, A. A., ... & Johnson, S. K. (2018). The Nutritional and Phytochemical Composition of the Indigenous Australian Pindan Walnut (Terminalia cunninghamii) Kernels. Plant Foods for Human Nutrition, In Press.

Index

271

Index

Index

Index

Index

vitamin C, 4, 24, 28,
  103, 136–137, 210
vitamin D, 103–104
vitamin E, 23
vitamin K1, 104
vitamin K2, 104
vitamins, 100–104

W

Warragul greens,
  220–221
water spinach, 221
watercress, 192–193
watermelon, 193
wattle seeds, 221–222
weight gain, 47
weight management,
  44–51, 114, 182, 227
    and grapefruit, 152
white blood cells, 32,
  38

Z

zeaxanthin, 3, 25, 28,
  86–90, 142, 158, 177
zingerone, 148–149

Phytochemicals

Help prevent cancer

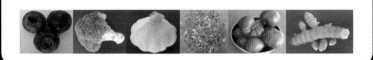

Help prevent cardiovascular disease

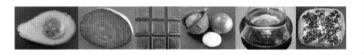

Help prevent dementia & relieve depression

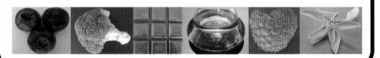

Maintain healthy eyes

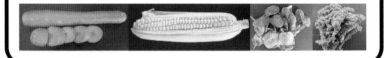

Help relieve inflammatory pain

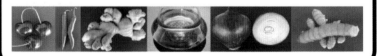